Mashed Potatoes and Gravy

A Woman's Journal through Surviving Cancer

BARBARA MADDOX

iUniverse, Inc.
New York Bloomington

iUniverse books may be ordered through booksellers or by contacting:

iUniverse
1663 Liberty Drive
Bloomington, IN 47403
www.iuniverse.com
1-800-Authors (1-800-288-4677)

ISBN: 978-1-4502-1868-9 (sc)
ISBN: 978-1-4502-1870-2 (dj)
ISBN: 978-1-4502-1869-6 (ebook)

Printed in the United States of America

iUniverse rev. date: 03/23/2010

For Chris

Cure sometimes, treat often, comfort always.
—Hippocrates

Contents

Introduction   xi

Cycle One: Shining a Light   1

Cycle Two: Finding Comforts   29

Cycle Three: The Universe Is Calling   69

Cycle Four: Breaking Spirit   93

Cycle Five: Balancing Act   121

Cycle Six: Being Human   139

Cycle Seven: Tipping Point   159

Cycle Eight: Clawing Out   183

Post-Treatment: A New Beginning   195

Introduction

I collapsed in my sister's arms that night in June, sobbing uncontrollably. I hung on to her for dear life, afraid to look around my own house, afraid to face the path that lay ahead of me—a journey through months of aggressive chemotherapy and a fight to beat a stage IV cancer diagnosis. I had just spent four days in the hospital, where I'd smiled lightheartedly, joking with the doctors and nurses and my visitors. I bravely faced each day in their care, being prodded, tested, having biopsies of a lymph node and my bone marrow, and getting five pints of blood infused into my veins, making me feel more alive than I had felt for months. It was easy there; people were tending to me, checking on me every hour, watching over me, bringing me cards and flowers, showering me in warmth and love and support. Then I was discharged. Riding in the car next to my husband, I could feel my stomach tighten with each mile we traveled toward our house, just minutes away from all that flurry and surreal experience of the last few days. My hands gripped at the car seat and the door handle. At home, who was going to watch over me? It was this stark reality that hit me square in the face, and I realized the battle was mine and mine alone.

My sister and her husband and my brother followed us home. I got out of the car and walked into my house, my wonderful home—how I had missed it. But it didn't feel welcoming. I'd barely taken ten steps inside when the rush of reality was too great, too frightening, and I turned, thinking I might faint. And thank goodness my sister was behind me. I went limp, the full weight of my body being held up by her nurturing love, and my sobs were like nothing I had ever heard, a gut-wrenching emotional release of pent-up fear. "Oh, my God," I cried, "I am *so* scared." The meltdown caught my siblings and my husband by surprise—there was no sign of this weakness in the months prior as I soldiered on searching for the answers to my failing health, nor in the hospital when I first learned of the cancer diagnosis. My strength and positive mental spirit had amazed everyone. I had them fooled. Hell, I'd fooled myself.

Millions have faced a similar health challenge and survived. Yet even that realization offers minimal comfort when you are the one going through it. Millions have died fighting cancer—now, that fact is what you cling to and think of every night. It was the security blanket I held and nurtured as I fell asleep each night throughout the journey. I always thought of those who fought the battle and lost. I was going to survive in their name. I wore this like a badge of honor.

My husband was the glue. No doubt about it. We had been married a little more than two years when cancer struck, and as I reflect upon this now, his entrée into my life was predestined and came just when I needed it most. During the first couple of days we were in the hospital, we spent much of our time talking on the phone and updating family and friends on my status. He realized that an online Web page would make our lives easier by allowing us to communicate more timely and more fully with our inner circle of loved ones versus the exhausting parade of phone calls and e-mail retelling the same story over and over.

There are a few very good Web services that offer online communication sites to cancer patients for free. We researched a couple of them and thought they would be quite useful. Fortunately for us, I have a best friend who is a marketing genius and Web designer. She designed a custom Web page for me, and it literally transformed my journey and my life. Not only did journaling about my experience provide me the necessary mental therapy to get through the daily grind of grueling treatments and nagging side effects, it served as the central communication piece to friends and family. And it reignited my love for writing, which eventually redirected my career away from the corporate world.

These pages contain the entries I wrote on my Web page during my treatments. I journaled two to four times per week, dating each entry like a diary. Months later, when the prodding from family and friends to publish these writings as a book became a goal worth pursuing, I reviewed the piece in its entirety and realized that the actual dates didn't really mean much. Furthermore, I realized each entry had, for the most part, a theme, which essentially influenced the subtitles that name each section. These sections (entries) are grouped into nine parts, congruent with my eight rounds of chemo and the post-treatment. And although there are some entries where it appears I jump around a variety of topics, I hope that illustrates some of the randomness that goes on in a chemo-hazed brain, under the influence of many (prescription) drugs.

One aspect of my Web page that is not captured here was a medical update section. This portion of the site explained in more medical terms the various results of blood tests, procedures, exams, and doctor visits throughout my treatment plan. For those in my support network who were interested in those gory details, this clinical point of view was helpful. My journal writings were more free-form expression where I didn't focus very much on medical jargon. So, throughout the book, a reader not familiar with chemotherapy might have a question or two about the importance of blood and the respective counts of both red and white cells. I'll offer a brief summary here.

In short, chemo drugs kill cells—good and bad. While there are some drugs that specifically target abnormal cells, the world of medicine is not yet perfected to be discriminating enough to root out only cancer cells. Chemotherapy is designed to attack cells in a state of change (whether that be newly forming, developing, or dying stages). Blood is one of the fastest-reproducing cells in the body. Cancer cells, generally speaking, also reproduce at a rapid rate. Chemotherapy attacks these fast-producing cells, also referred to as turnover cells. Thus, the assault on cancer cells and blood—and the linings of the mouth and digestive tract, as these areas also have cells with quicker turnover cycles.

Blood, of course, is your lifeline, carrying oxygen throughout your body (through the red cells) and providing clotting abilities (through the platelets), as well as providing vital infection-fighting properties (through the white cells). For patients on chemotherapy, blood counts are taken often as a way to measure a couple of things: how well one is progressing throughout treatment against the disease and if those counts are strong enough to proceed with treatment. Counts too low can suspend or delay treatment. It is a delicate balancing act, as delaying treatment in some cases means the cancer cells may continue to multiply, which could impact treatability and curability rates. In order to keep as close to the scheduled treatment plan as possible, doctors prescribe drugs that promote growth of white and red cells to maintain the levels necessary for chemotherapy. Infusions of packed red cells and platelets become necessary when these growth drugs are ineffective or too slow. For the white cells, however, there is no infusion remedy to increase their count. Only a drug or the body's own production can impact white cells.

Hodgkin's lymphoma is a blood disease, and like all lymphomas, a cancer of the lymphatic system. This system filters the body's blood and supports the immune system (the body's defense against infection). Hodgkin's is a very treatable and potentially curable disease, generally more so than other non-Hodgkin's lymphomas. Unfortunately, there has been a rise in lymphomas over the past few years, according to recent cancer reports. The Leukemia & Lymphoma Society (LLS) reports that an estimated 74,490 persons living in the United States in 2009 will be diagnosed with lymphoma, of which 8,510 diagnoses will be Hodgkin's disease[1]. Hodgkin's is a cancer that strikes the young—teenagers and young adults in their twenties—and men more than women. It also afflicts older adults who are in their sixties to seventies. I was forty-three when I was diagnosed, not quite the typical candidate. The staging of the disease depends on its progress from one lymph node, to multiple nodes, to the organs. In my case, I had cancer cells in multiple nodes as well as an organ—my bone marrow—which put my diagnosis in stage IV. Additionally, some of the symptoms I experienced, particularly the night sweats, added a "type B" onto that diagnosis, which essentially meant I was in the worst possible scenario for the disease. Thankfully, the survivability and curability rates, even at my age and stage level, were all in my favor.

I was equally lucky with the medical staff tending to my care and the medical facilities where I was treated. Sky Ridge Medical Center is a state-of-the-art facility, built within the last decade and located just a few minutes from my (then) home in Parker, Colorado. Additionally, the hematologist to whom I was referred was located right next door to the hospital. His practice has been noted as one of the top oncology offices in the state. They operate another location about twenty-five minutes away on Hampden Avenue, which is where I sometimes received my treatments. The infusion center at Sky Ridge was also a place I visited

---

1   The Leukemia & Lymphoma Society, Disease Information > Lymphoma, www.leukemia-lymphoma.org/all_page?item_id=7030.

often, where I received most of the twenty-plus pints of blood and several units of platelets throughout my treatment.

This book is my journey through chemotherapy to cancer survivorship. It's an accounting of my thoughts, emotions, physical state, and my relationships with family, friends, and the universe. You'll find no how-to instructions, undiscovered remedies, or far-flung advice. It's just my story, and one that I hope offers some solace and comfort, particularly for those facing a similar life challenge—like having an old friend along for the ride. Beyond that, it's a simple narrative, not uncommon to many, of managing through a real-life trauma with some self-discovery along the way. Family, friends, food, and good humor provided much relief in the trying times. Those comforts were a blessing, like being wrapped in a soft blanket on a cold night, snuggled next to a warm fire with a good book, sipping a cup of tea or eating a plateful of mashed potatoes and gravy.

CYCLE ONE

Shining a Light

The Beginning
June 2008

Day one of chemotherapy. I'm sitting in the doctor's office as I write this, getting a dose of one of the many chemo drugs I will receive intravenously. I have a port in my chest that was surgically inserted last Friday. The site is still a little sore and so swollen that the nurse's first attempt to access the port with an IV needle was very difficult. It hurt, the pain a shock to my system. I hyperventilated and felt like I was going to faint. I couldn't get my breath under control as fear gripped my body and I started sobbing. Reality was sinking in. Another nurse came over to help calm me. After about twenty minutes, they attempted the needle insertion again—this time successfully—*and so the journey begins.*

So far today, I've had two drugs intravenously—one for nausea, the other a steroid to help the nausea medication. As I continue to write, I'm currently receiving drug number three, which is one of the chemo drugs. I'll get three more through the IV before I leave today. By mouth, I have already taken a different drug for nausea and two other chemo drugs. One of the oral chemo drugs is actually a steroid, prednisone. This little pill, at the dosage I'm taking, will cause all sorts of wonderful symptoms like water retention and puffiness in the face, weight gain, and insomnia. I'll have fourteen days of this special pill. The other oral chemo drug is procarbazine, which I'll take for seven days. I get to come back to the doctor's office the next two days, rest four days at home, and then report back for two consecutive days next week. A total of five out of nine days that I'll get poked in the chest. Then a week off to recoup and we start the routine all over again.

I'm not the first to go through this, nor will I be the last. The treatments sound daunting, but frankly, I welcome them. All I want to do is kick this thing and start the second half of my life 100 percent healthy. I expect the chemotherapy to do its job, and I will do my job of tending to my mental and spiritual side, and tough it out through the rough days ahead.

✳ ✳ ✳

Two days of treatment and I am kind of surprised that I am still feeling *okay*. I definitely feel like I have drugs flowing through me, but I have experienced nothing yet of the horrible side effects. They tell me to expect that by the weekend. My mom will stay with me for a few days. There is nothing like the comfort of your mom squeezing your hand and holding back your hair while you puke in a bucket.

Speaking of hair, I did get my long mane chopped off this past weekend prior to starting my chemotherapy treatment. Yes, my brown and golden tresses are gone—and in their place is a pretty sassy-looking bob. I must say, I truly dig it. I decided to take charge and go short now. Better to pull out clumps of short hair than long hair—less traumatic, ya know?

Day two of the first cycle is in the books, only three hours in the doctor's office (versus seven yesterday). I have great confidence in the medical team treating me. My doctor is extremely thorough; the nurses are caring and definitely in your camp. And the biggest support at my side is my husband. Chris has been absolutely amazing. The care and concern he has shown for me demonstrates the depth of his love for me. How very lucky I am.

My Sanctuary

After three days of chemo at the doctor's office and one day at home to recoup, *so far, so good*. I thought I'd have my head in a bucket or over the toilet. I am tired for sure and have much discomfort in my belly area, but other than that, I am able to get around well and do things for myself.

What a comfort it is to have my mom here for a few days. She lives only across town and doesn't drive, so my brother dropped her off to stay with me. And although she is on oxygen, she wants to help so much, bless her heart. You should see us—I'm busy trying to make sure she's comfortable, while she's trying to comfort me. She can get around pretty easily; she is feisty—that's where I get my spirit. (She claims we're so different, but we're much more alike than she would ever admit.) My other siblings were here as well today. I am being well cared for.

You should see the sanctuary my husband has built for me in the little sitting room of our master bedroom. It is awesome. Chris is a mighty good project manager, and I and my plight have become Project Barb. He envisioned this space—a calming, working retreat—without my input, but he knew such a place would make life simpler for me, and he also knew I would not ask for the trouble. And the trouble people have gone through for me is heartwarming. Chris is a great visionary but needs a team around him, being more of a director and leader and less of an expert in things such as electronics, interior design, and the operation of certain hand tools. I have a new flat-screen TV on the wall, which I can also use as a computer monitor. My brother-in-law, Ken, wired the room, and my brother Michael set up my remote keyboard and mouse. I have a handsome leather chaise lounge, which will serve as my nap couch, my television-viewing couch, and my reading and journaling couch. My friend Tami helped me decorate with pictures and candles to bring some warmth to the room. I must admit, I feel a little spoiled, but that's okay, isn't it?

I cannot find the words to express what I am feeling in my heart for people rallying to my side. One of my dear friends, Jackie, put together a custom Web site where I can post medical updates and, more importantly, journal about my experiences. Another idea born in that splendid mind of my husband's. The Saturday after I was released from the hospital, Chris organized a planning meeting, which included my sister Jeanette, brother Michael, and good friends Alex and Tami. Together they launched Project Barb and have made my transition to this journey comfortable and worry-free, to my most delightful surprise. My sister has been my champion and is managing online calendars for meals and my medical appointments. She is so thankful for the help of Alex, who has rallied the BOTS girls, my book-club girlfriends, to assist with Project Me. (BOTS is "Books on the Side," appropriately named because we frankly do not always read the chosen book—if one is even chosen—so the reading of books falls to the side, as we prefer to enjoy each other's company and drink much wine.)

Okay, I'm tired now. Gotta go.

Earthly Angels
July 2008

I am so excited to be through *day eight* of chemo treatments! No more chemo drugs until my second cycle begins in two weeks. While I still have six more days of steroids to complete this round, I have come out of this first chemo cycle *a-okay!* I am feeling much weakness, to be sure, and some discomfort with nausea and constipation, but overall, I am not too beat up. Wow!

Oh, and then there were the psychedelic dreams I had the other night. I dreamed all night I was pregnant and trying to save the baby from cancer! And I was so tired in the dream; I just wanted to lie down anywhere to rest. At one point, I was sleeping on the pavement in front of Wal-Mart. Seriously. And two small, black homeless children were huddled up with me trying to keep warm. Yeah, those kinds of psychedelic dreams.

I truly cannot believe this experience. I am met with pleasant surprises every day. Today at the doctor's office while I was receiving chemo, I was seated next to a younger girl receiving iron supplements intravenously. We looked at each other with a nod of acknowledgement, as if to silently say "There's someone young like me." We struck up a conversation, and it turns out she's much younger than me. Twenty-six, to be exact. And she's been battling serious health issues since she was thirteen, half of her life.

Her history started in 1995 with thyroid cancer. Since then, she has had multiple chemotherapy sessions, 75 percent of her small intestines removed, and a host of other tumors and ailments. But she did not seem deterred or deflated by her misfortunes and a life sentence of health challenges. I marveled at this young, beautiful girl who had the face of an angel. This is her life, and she openly shared with me her story. I felt anchored by her, supported and lifted. She has grown up in Colorado and has only her mother, who looks after her. I thought about my situation and how blessed I am to have such an incredible, deep network of family and friends, and my heart ached for her. But she did not know the difference.

Through her sharing, *she* comforted *me*. And when she left, I cried, having just been touched by an angel. I hope I see her again soon. I have a feeling I will meet many more earthly angels in the coming days.

* * *

Okay, today my butt is kicked. I didn't sleep well last night. I got up very early this morning and wrote e-mails and did a few things around the house—probably not the best thing to do after a sleepless night. The chemo drugs from yesterday had me feverish. My intestines feel like they're turned inside out. But I am resting well now.

The launch for my Web site looks like a success, with already so many wonderful posts from friends and family! These messages of love and hope truly stir in me the healing power to get me through this challenge.

Been thinking a lot about how the universe opens up and gives you just about what you need and can handle. I'll write more on the topic at a later time. Shutting my eyes for now.

Crazy, Yes—Sexy, No

Happy Independence Day. A good day to celebrate independence from cancer. That is my goal. I just finished watching the documentary *Crazy, Sexy, Cancer*. My brother loaned me the DVD a couple of weeks ago, and it has taken me several days before I could watch it. I've noticed that it does take me some time to turn my attention to books, magazines, and any other types of information given to me on the topic of cancer. There is a point where your mind bubbles and protects you from having too much information. And then there's the added benefit of having "chemo brain," which causes lapses in concentration and memory. The nurses tell me this will improve after treatment. I didn't think I was too much of an airhead before, but then again … The chemo is also affecting my vision. Now, this sucks. Two weeks before this whole wonderful journey began, I invested in a sassy-looking pair of Versace glasses. (Can you say "bling-bling"?) Things are a little blurry with or without glasses. This should subside after treatment as well.

So, back to the DVD—it was a great documentary. I cried, I laughed, I was inspired by the story of a young woman facing an incurable cancer. Incurability is not something I face, but I definitely related to her journey. Chris was inspired as well. He wants to buy a Vita-Mix blender tomorrow to start juicing and drinking healthy concoctions like the woman in the documentary. I'm not quite there yet. Trying to find the right balance of food and nutrition is tricky. I have an appetite again thanks to the steroid, but the gas pain is quite unpleasant.

I am a walking pharmacy. Drugs, anyone? I have two new BFFs: Ambien, which I call Amber, and Vicodin, which I nicknamed Vicky. Amber helps me sleep; Vicky takes away the pain. I don't have to reach for Vicky much at all, but I did tonight. The shot I got in my arm yesterday to stimulate white blood cell production is creating some pain in the bones of my lower back—a side effect. Should sleep like a baby tonight with my two BFFs, hopefully sans freaky dreams.

Don't Be a Doormat

Anger. It finally hit me Friday, late in the night—or one in the morning, to be exact—as I was doing some Web surfing for more information about my actual disease. I'm in an advanced stage of Hodgkin's. Did I need to be here? All my doctor visits came flooding back to me, and I went round and round in my head with the conversations and check-ups I had since the beginning of the year. Here on my chaise lounge in the middle of the night, my symptoms were being spelled out to me in black and white on the various lymphoma Web sites—why did my family doctor try to explain them away? I also went back and read the journal entries in the medical update section on my Web page, the first one that detailed my months of ill health. It's there in black and white, too. Sure, each of my symptoms can be related to another, less serious illness, but seeing them grouped all together *should* have moved my doctor in the direction of at least considering lymphoma. *It's all right there!* I felt my blood pressure rise, and I got pretty pissed off because seven months later, I'm in stage IV. Maybe I was in an earlier stage back in January when I started seeing that doctor; who knows? And even though the later stage is still treatable and potentially curable, the complication and relapse rates are higher, and I am receiving very aggressive chemotherapy because of the disease's progress.

Some of my family and friends are probably thinking, "It's about time she's mad. How could she not be angry that her doctor missed the boat?" Yeah, I was definitely trying to be a little too understanding of the position my family doctor was in—having to find out her patient of seven months ended up in the ER because she failed to run the proper tests. She even visited me in the hospital, the day after I went to the emergency room, still trying to explain her way out of why we didn't go down this path earlier, and why the enlarged lymph nodes that were detected on a chest CT scan (that was finally ordered by the ER doctor) could be related to other issues, such as mono (which I had in February, one of the few things she diagnosed correctly), and that mono can lead to some more severe infections and lupus is still a possibility; and so you see, don't think that cancer is necessarily going to be the diagnosis; I don't want you to worry. She needed to stop while she was ahead. I know in my heart she had the best intentions for me—our doctors should and do. But, along with this realization of being totally pissed off comes a recognition of responsibility—*my* responsibility, that I have to push for the right answers. When I had tried to self-diagnose my illness earlier in the year, scanning the Internet for answers to my symptoms, I distinctly remember dismissing the word lymphoma when it came up once during my research. *No way I have cancer,* I told myself. It's not in my family—we have a history of high blood pressure and heart disease. So even I didn't want to broach the topic of cancer with my family doctor, but shouldn't she have known?

My advice to anyone is this: if you are ill and not improving or only marginally improving, and the symptoms start to become part of your routine and something you just live with—push for answers. Become informed. You have to take charge of your health and not be afraid of the answers. Knowledge is freedom.

The Family Circle

Family. Unbelievable support and undeniable strength. I don't know where I would be without my siblings. We are an emotional bunch. My sister and two brothers are my anchors. They are guiding this vessel of mine, nurturing it, keeping me buoyant, and making me laugh and cry. My sister, Jeanette, is the oldest, followed by Rick, then me and Michael. In age, we are forty-five, forty-four, forty-three, and forty-two. That's right, only one year separates one sibling from the next. Mom and Dad were quite busy making this unique, close set of kids. We are so different and so alike, each of us. My mother is Filipina, first generation. We don't know that side of our family except through stories from Mom. It was my father and his side of the family that really helped to nurture the closeness I share with my siblings today.

My father passed away eight summers ago. We were very close. I was (still am) the quintessential daddy's little girl. Every year since I can remember, there has been a family reunion on my dad's side of the family back East. As we were growing up, these reunions were special to me and my siblings, even though we only attended a handful of them throughout the years. When my father passed away in 2000, his brothers and sisters came to visit him on his deathbed and stayed to attend the funeral service. They were like a huge bear hug to us during that sad time. We attended the reunion the very next year, and it was one filled with high emotion and memories—a touching tribute to my father. Since that reunion, our Colorado clan had not attended another until last year, when the patriarch of Dad's family, his brother Harold, passed away. There was no way we were going to miss that reunion and the opportunity to offer back to Uncle Harold's family the same love and support they had given us years ago when my father died.

The dynamic of these reunions has changed over the years. We are older, more mature; the former kids are now parents of their own, and some are even very young grandparents! We have lost husbands, fathers, sons, grandmothers, and great-grandmothers. We have figured out (and for the most part, accepted) that not everyone shares the same beliefs or lifestyles. But we are all family and follow that tribal tradition of caring for your own, loving each other no matter what. During last year's reunion, we were so touched by the uplifting and moving memorial service for my Uncle Harold. This event seemed to strongly reconnect our Colorado contingent to the rest of Dad's family. My siblings and I decided right then and there that we would do our best each year to attend the reunion, wherever the family planned to hold it.

This year's reunion is scheduled to take place in two and half weeks. Those of us in Colorado (fifteen in all) had been planning to attend. Then my illness struck. I was still hopeful that Chris and I would be able to travel, but after going through one round of chemo, it seemed my energy level would not permit me to attend. This was a major disappointment for me, but the right decision, particularly since the second round of chemo starts that very week.

What I didn't realize was that the rest of the Colorado gang was struggling with the same decision of whether or not to go *because of me*. My sister Jeanette and brother Rick were visiting this weekend, when I first learned they were contemplating not going. My immediate response upon hearing this news was, "No way. That would piss me off!" I didn't want this stupid disease to screw up everyone else's life. Plus, I thought it would be cathartic for them to be with Dad's family, away from the craziness that having cancer renders you to. My encouraging them to still go only made them struggle more. What was going on? Rick finally said that he didn't want to go away and come back to find that he hadn't been around to offer his support while his baby sister went through some change like my hair falling out completely. My sister added that they wouldn't be enjoying themselves very much, as all their thoughts would be on me back home. It just didn't make any sense to them that they be anywhere else except with me. I was floored. *Really? You care about me that much?*

It never occurred to me that this was weighing so heavy on their minds. And when I finally accepted the full force of unconditional love being thrown at me, *they* were so relieved. Trapped in my own regret for deciding to forgo this year's reunion, I did not recognize how much my not being there would impact their experience. "There's next year," Jeanette said, "when we all will be together—100 percent healthy." And so the emotions flowed and so did our tears. These beautiful siblings of mine are my lifeline. And now there's nowhere else they'd rather be than right by my side. What better feeling is there?

Simple Joys

Okay, time for a little levity. Life has slowed down quite a bit the last month, giving me a chance to find new daily joys. For instance, finding the right over-the-counter drug for gas pain is now nirvana. And I have read that chewing each bite fifty times at meals is recommended to aid digestion. Did you know that? Try it. I never quite get to fifty, but after thirty or forty chews, the stuff liquefies in your mouth. I actually have found food much more flavorful and enjoyable that way.

I am a student in Basic Training for Health 101—all the things they should teach you about health and nutrition, but never did. I've got four or five books open all around me at one time. I feel like I'm back in school, only this time, it's the school of life. And I'm learning so much.

So returning to my list of newly found simple joys (and not necessarily in any order of importance): hugs from my niece, Elsa; loose stools; beautiful, heart-tugging posts on my Web page; funny, hysterical posts on my Web page; a warm sitz bath for hemorrhoids; visits from friends; breaking a sweat from a leisurely thirty-minute walk; sleeping four straight hours; ice cream cake; water; a healing hangnail; veggie omelets; chocolate; my husband's sweet kisses on the top of my head; stopping a nosebleed; a great CD; rinsing with a solution of baking soda and water to soothe mouth sores; and, of course, all the love and well-wishes from everyone.

I've got one more day of steroids and then I'm off treatment until next Tuesday. That's a great joy. I have blood work tomorrow—hope my counts are good.

Drugs and More Drugs

I am the Bionic Woman (some days "Plutonium" Woman). While you cannot put a price tag on one's life, I am quickly finding out what it means to have good insurance coverage. Thankfully, I have it and it's good. So, I am bionic, or surely worth six million dollars, because every little chemo drug is sooooo ultra-expensive, and every little shot, like the one I received today, is like putting a diamond in my veins.

I had a complete blood count done again today. With the cancer impacting my bone marrow, checking blood counts will become a weekly routine. I now have two new shots to add to my BFF list of drugs (remember Amber and Vicky?). Someone actually asked me the other day what BFF meant. Hello? Best Friends Forever. Okay, so the two new shots are Neulasta and Procrit. Neulasta is the growth drug for creating white blood cells. I'll call her Nesta. Procrit promotes red blood cell production. I'll call her Prudy (a stretch, but can't think of a closer chick name).

Unlike the chemo drugs, which I can't quite elevate to BFF status because they make me so sick, Nesta and Prudy should help keep my blood counts where they need to be so I can continue on with the chemo treatments. They are an expensive pair. Nesta is $2,500 a pop and Prudy $4,000! Shocking, I know, but good-quality insurance is happy to pick up the tab. Frankly, a designer bag from Dolce & Gabbana would be cheaper but may not give me quite the lift I need. Nesta did her job from her last week's injection; my white blood cell counts are higher. Prudy needs to give me some help, because my red blood cell count is low and making me very, very tired. Getting a shot of Prudy means I may not need a blood transfusion. I am hoping she kicks in soon, because I have a lot more to write and have been able to do nothing except take naps all day. I had started to take morning walks, but the nurses told me not to do that for a few days with my blood count so low. Take it easy.

Oh, one last thing about Nesta and Prudy before my chemo brain shuts down for the night. Chris and I asked the nurse why they're so expensive. She explained that these drugs are lab generated, which makes them costly to produce. Neulasta is derived from E. coli. That's right, folks, I am getting an injection of E. coli in such high amounts that my body has no choice but to kick white blood cell production into gear. And Procrit comes from a gerbil's ovaries. Something in that ovary does something else in your kidney, which tells the bone marrow to produce hemoglobin. E. coli and a rodent's ovary *in my body*. The amazing world of medicine.

So, as if my having cancer isn't already a life-altering experience, Chris has taken a new job in the midst of all of this craziness. It is a good thing, and I am very proud of my hubby. It was a tough decision for him—for us—given the circumstances. But it made sense, in that it is a wonderful opportunity, a director-level position, and taps into the very essence of his strong skill sets of project management and just basically making shit happen. He will make more dough (yay!) and be home based (yay, yay!). This will provide us some flexibility and relief while I recover and will allow me that time to do so free of any nagging thoughts about finances.

Remember that universe opening up and giving you just what you need at the right time? Chris and I have been feeling that kind of ethereal support for the past month. It's a very strange thing to say as you face down cancer, but we know there are only good things on our horizon, despite what looks like big hurdles. We're ready to face these challenges together, and I'll get through anything with my awesome husband by my side.

With the new job, Chris will be quite preoccupied. There will be travel involved, and he was a little hesitant to accept the position because of it. So, we've tapped into that wonderful family-friend network of ours to ensure there are plenty of folks ready to watch over me while he embarks on this new career. My family is not going to the reunion, and my sister and brother have vacation time they'll be spending with me. Chris's mom is coming out for two weeks in August. And we have a host of friends all around us. We are so very blessed, humbled, speechless when it comes to the support network we have. Thank you, Universe.

Temporary Phases

It's here. The scary bad-hair day. It's falling out. I had read about this moment in the many reference books I have open at any one time. Over the last week, single strands of my hair had been shedding here and there—nothing alarming. My scalp had been tingling for days, feeling like it was having its own out-of-body experience, seemingly lifting from my head. *Any day*, was my thought, *there will be more and I will handle it—you know it's coming*. Nearly a foot of hair was cut down to that sassy bob to avoid a tangled, matted mess. So, I thought I was prepared. I wasn't.

There I was this morning in the shower gently shampooing my hair, and as I pulled away my hand, clumps of hair stuck to my fingers. My heart stopped. I stood there staring at the thick, wet, brown ropes of my old self in my palm. The tears flowed. I felt so alone, so vulnerable, so sad at that moment. I didn't move for what seemed an eternity, until slowly, I touched my head to rinse the rest of the shampoo, and more clumps pulled away from my scalp. I just sobbed in silence, trying to be as gentle as possible, to preserve the remaining shafts. Out of the shower, the shedding continued as I dried and styled what hair was left. Thankfully, I have a thick head of hair and what I lost this morning was proportionate, so the remainder still maintains its basic shape. But having this much hair also means it's going to be a messy next few days as this mop continues to fall out in pieces.

As it happens, I had an appointment on this very day to meet with a lady who custom-fits wigs for cancer patients. I had called Linda's Boutique the day before to ask for directions, thinking I could just drop in to check out the selection. The voice on the other end of the phone told me that I needed an appointment; I could not just "drop in"—there was a *process* to what she did. I asked her if she was Linda. "No. My name is Mary." There is no Linda at Linda's Boutique. So I went ahead and made an appointment. *This should be interesting*, I thought.

Chris came with me, as Mary (not Linda) recommended I bring someone for support. After I'd pulled myself together from this morning's tragic shedding event, we headed down to Linda's Boutique for the *process* of being fitted for a wig. Stepping into the shop was like taking a step back in time. The air was old and stale, and there was big-band-era music playing in the background. I looked around for the transistor radio just to be sure, but I didn't see one. On display throughout the boutique were all kinds of colorful shapes and sizes of hats, with some wigs and scarves sprinkled throughout. The shop felt old, but there was a comfort in that oldness—like a wise soul had lived there for eons. Out comes Mary, a thin woman in her sixties, with big, warm, brown eyes and shoulder-length hair and a smile that immediately put me at ease. She knew what I was going through.

Mary has been working with cancer patients for years, helping them transition to the temporary status of the hairless. And it was a *process* working with her—first find the right wig color to complement the face, she explained, and once we find the right color, she then orders that wig and I come back for a fitting and have it styled any way I like. She took time to show me how to wear scarves and what types of hats are good for the shape of my face. She gave me all kinds of advice, not just about head fashion but also about what side effects to expect from chemo and the different remedies her past clients have used. And she was full of stories and words of encouragement. Her daughter had Hodgkin's lymphoma nearly twenty years ago and is cancer-free. Her husband was diagnosed with a different cancer two and a half years ago and, while it sounded as if he had been struggling with his disease, she focused only on his positive outlook. Mary definitely chose to see the glass as half full. She extended herself for nearly two hours to me, not receiving a dime or commitment that I would purchase anything—in fact, she discouraged me from getting too many hats or scarves, as she said I'd end up wearing a couple of favorite pieces, so don't waste money. It was a good experience.

As I was leaving, Mary handed me hair nets to wear overnight to capture the hair that will continue to shed. But more than a hair net, she threw me a safety net and reminded me that this health-challenged, hairless phase of my life is only temporary.

✳ ✳ ✳

Just a quick update on how I've been feeling. The last two days have been difficult; I can definitely feel the low red-blood counts affecting me. I am almost as weak as I felt when I went to the emergency room five weeks ago. My doctor and nurses had told me to expect this. I'm taking it as easy as I can. My nose is giving me fits—chemo drip, they call it. I popped some Claritin, which should help dry that up. I have a throbbing sinus headache. Took Tylenol for that. Physically, I'm whipped, but mentally, I am very strong. The Procrit shot (Prudy) should be lifting my counts this weekend, I hope, and I'll get some extra energy.

Out of the Darkness

Today, for a couple of reasons, I'm going to chronicle the last several months of searching for an answer for my health issues: first, to stop dwelling on it and move on, and second, to help anyone else who may be having a similar experience recognize earlier than I did when to take more aggressive action.

September of 2007 is when I noticed a drop in my energy level and an overall feeling of the "blahs." I work in the building-products industry, and business had been declining at that point for several months, creating lots of stress. Our company was trying to define and refine its culture, and we were going through layoffs and job restructuring, putting more workload on the staff that remained. At the time, I had been with the company for nine years, had built a good reputation, and enjoyed the customers, employees, and the type of business I handled. Throughout my career, I had experienced great personal success and progress and survived several downturns in the business cycles when we had to tighten our belts and lay off many fellow employees. I'd been through it all before, but for some reason, this particular downtrend had more impact on my state of mind. I was beginning to feel quite disconnected from the direction the company was heading, which seemed to focus less on *human* capital and more on *making* capital for our executive managers and shareholders. People all around me were staking out their own turf and thrusting forth their personal agendas; there was a lot of chest-beating going on, and sadly, too much backstabbing. Outwardly, I was playing the game; inwardly, it was wreaking havoc on my psyche.

It was during this latest downturn that I started experiencing what I believed to be stress-related muscle tension and headaches. I was already seeing a chiropractor, and I began massage therapy in his office on a weekly basis. My muscles were knotted up in my back and neck, and the massages were offering some temporary relief. In October of 2007,

I noticed a hard knot on my neck, above my right clavicle. This alarmed me; it hadn't been there before. I pointed it out to the masseuse one day at the chiropractor's office. She felt the area and determined it wasn't muscular; she said to have the chiropractor check it out. He did and told me not to be alarmed and that if it was still there in a week to have it examined by a medical doctor. Sometimes, he explained, our bodies are trying to get rid of infection and stress, and our lymph nodes respond to that. It went away after a couple of days, and I didn't think about it again, until months later.

I continued to have weekly massages and went about my life. Work stress and gamesmanship persisted, and we had a bigger layoff toward the end of October. November seemed to quiet a little on the work front, but I started to notice some gradual weight loss. I had been spending most of my waking hours at the office or traveling on business and didn't make time for workouts at the gym. So it was odd that I was losing weight. I also developed a very mild cough. I could feel a tickling sensation under my sternum that wasn't bothersome, it just made me cough on occasion. This light cough stayed with me for several weeks.

Something else was happening that I did not relate to a poor health issue at the time—night sweats. I remember one evening at a friend's house while we were playing cards, I mentioned that I started having night sweats. I would wake up with my neck and chest soaked in sweat. My girlfriend said to me, "Welcome to the forties!" So I didn't think anything of it, other than my own body was possibly experiencing hormonal changes.

Throughout the holidays, this general feeling of the blahs continued, accompanied by a low energy level, neck and muscle tightness, the cough, a gradual decline in weight, and a new symptom: loss of appetite. The loss of appetite was interesting. I was hungry at the right times, and when I made food, I wanted to eat it. But as soon as I took a couple of bites, I felt full or just lost interest in the food altogether. From the beginning of November through Christmas, I dropped seven pounds. Generally, I gain a few pounds, as do many people around the holidays. Again, I thought possibly my body was off due to changing hormone levels. I decided to seek out a doctor and scheduled an appointment on New Year's Eve, December 31, 2007.

I remember my method for selecting a doctor. I wanted a female, close to my work or home, and someone who was young versus old. I figured that a doctor who'd been in practice a few short years may have kept more current with the latest medical developments and would be more in tune with the medical needs of a woman similar in age—something I now believe was a flaw in my thinking, because ultimately what I needed was someone with more experience in diagnosing serious illness.

At the first visit with this young family doctor, I explained all my troubling symptoms. My main concern was the fatigue and the neck and muscle pain. I explained to her what I did for a living, the work stress I had been experiencing, the cough and slight tightness in my chest that made me cough. I did not tell her about the swollen lymph node I had in October—I had forgotten about it. I told her that Chris had been sick with a bad cold in November and that's when I noticed the scratchiness in my throat, but weeks later I still had it. She gave me a bronchodilator in the office to open up my passages, which gave me some relief. She checked my vitals; my blood pressure was a little elevated, but it didn't concern her. She concluded that possibly I had a very slight case of bronchitis, which can last for several weeks. She also mentioned the possibility that I was suffering from anxiety or depression. I balked at the depression suggestion. I didn't feel depressed. She gave me one prescription for an inhaler and another to see a physical therapist for my muscle tension. I was thrilled with that recommendation; I didn't know I could see someone medically for knotted muscles!

I started physical therapy right away. The initial examination pointed to poor posture. Chris would always admonish me for the way I sat at work (we worked at the same company—that's how we met), hunched over the computer, and it was also something my chiropractor had talked to me about. But rather than adjusting my spine, the physical therapist worked directly on the joints and muscles in my back and neck and did wonders! I finally felt some relief. He gave me tips on how to improve posture at work, which I implemented right away.

It was the first of the year, and I was as anxious as any New Year's resolution purist to get my health back on track and begin working out and being active again. I had missed being consistent with workouts for several months. At the end of January, Chris and I went skiing, which caused me to have a physical meltdown! The altitude affected me much more than normal, and I could only get down two ski runs before my legs gave out. I had to stop several times during the middle of each run to catch my breath and to relieve my quadriceps from cramping up completely. I was so dismayed and thought how pathetic I was for letting myself get so out of shape! The odd thing about the cramping and accompanying soreness was that it didn't feel like the reaction from a typical lactic-acid buildup from overworked muscles—rather, my muscles and joints ached as if I had the flu. And the fatigue I had been feeling worsened.

A couple of days later, I traveled on business. Although my legs were still feeling a flu-like ache, I managed this trip successfully, only to return home on that Thursday evening, bedridden from some kind of stomach bug I had caught somewhere along the way. On Friday morning, too exhausted to get out of bed, I called in sick. I was feeling better that Saturday, but then on Sunday—Super Bowl Sunday, to be exact—I felt another illness coming on, this time either the onset of a bad cold or the flu itself. Monday rolled around, and again, I could not get out of bed, suffering from heavy head congestion, muscle aches, and fever. Still sick on Tuesday, I made an appointment to see my doctor. We both suspected flu, right? Wrong. She tested me and I was negative for the flu. *Then what was this?* My doctor concluded that "What you have is viral, and there isn't anything to give you for it. I'm ordering you two to three more days of bed rest." I told her I wanted a complete physical, and she agreed and asked me to return in a couple weeks when my symptoms subsided. I was finally back at work on Friday, but still weak, and it would take me several more days to eventually shake off this viral infection.

It was now February 2008, and finally feeling over the recent bout of illness, I went on a couple of ski outings with Chris. One was just a day trip, and frustration visited me again. I had the same physical experience as I did the first time we went in January—out of shape, shortness of breath, incredible cramping in my legs. I was also feverish that night, and the night sweats, which had worsened during the viral bug episode, continued. In fact, the night sweats were so bad at this point, I was soaking my sheets and having to change out my pajamas twice during the night. I finally just started sleeping in between two thick towels. My sleep also was completely interrupted because of these episodes; all I could string together was a couple of hours at a time. I was lucky to get four or five hours of total sleep a night.

The next ski outing was in mid-February—a four-day weekend planned in Vail. This was an annual ski trip with friends from Atlanta.

Chris and I both looked forward to this outing, even though I was still struggling with my health issues. I lasted only one half-day on the slopes, again experiencing the same physical limitations as before. Nothing was improving.

At home, I started to do my own Internet surfing and entered all my symptoms on Web MD. The first thing that popped up was perimenopause. *Interesting*, I thought. Also on the list were thyroid disease, Epstein-Barr virus, lupus, lymphoma (I remember making a conscious decision to ignore any hints of cancer), and a host of other illnesses such as depression, anxiety, and flu.

It was the end of February when I returned to my doctor for a complete physical. I came to the meeting prepared with a written list of fourteen symptoms or health concerns that had plagued me the last few months; some had subsided but were still present to some degree. She noted my weight loss: ten pounds since my first visit with her two months ago on New Year's Eve. The list looked something like this: fatigue, neck and back muscle aches, headaches, night sweats, hot flashes, cough, sore lymph nodes (I was beginning to feel soreness in my armpits), shortness of breath, leg cramping, loss of appetite, shedding fifteen pounds since November. And at the bottom of the page, I wrote *depression*. She drew my blood, checked my lymph nodes, and performed other bodily checks. She told me that nothing from her physical touch on the various parts of my body seemed unusual. We then reviewed the list of symptoms in detail, along with my short history with her. She circled back around to depression—again. Even though I listed it last on my list, it was still a focus for her. I explained to her I was depressed because I had been feeling like shit for months. It was affecting my home and social life—all I had energy for was work. The blood work she ordered was extensive—a total of seven or eight items to check, including thyroid, hormone levels, lupus, inflammation, anemia. She said to me, "I think you're a healthy adult. What happens when all of these tests come back normal? Do you think you'd be ready to talk about depression?" She explained that depression is a disease in which sometimes you don't know what started first—the depression and then symptoms or vice versa. I listened to her, still not convinced that depression was the root cause of these symptoms. I told her I guessed we could have that conversation when the tests came back, but I truly in my gut did not feel depressed.

The following week, in early March, my doctor called me to tell me

I indeed was feeling real symptoms of an illness. I had a diagnosis: it was mono, or the Epstein-Barr virus. She explained that I was in what's called the convalescent stage of the illness, meaning it had moved on beyond the height of the typical symptoms (which I had felt as the flu), and things like the night sweats and fatigue could remain for two to four more weeks. She felt it explained the weight loss and loss of appetite as well as the soreness in my lymph nodes. I asked her when she thought this started. Unknown, she said, *But you've probably had it for several weeks at this point.* There was nothing she could give me for mono; it just had to run its course. I was relieved to have an answer. At the pit of my stomach, though, I wondered if that explained everything. She asked me to come back in three to four weeks for a follow-up and to run new blood tests to assure I was getting past the illness.

I didn't wait three to four weeks; I was actually back in her office two weeks later. Chris and I went to the mountains again to ski. I could sense that my husband was getting cabin fever because all my health issues had pretty much kept me sidelined from social activity, which meant he was cooped up with me. I had turned down numerous invitations for social gatherings, dinner out with friends, or family events—I just didn't have the energy, and my hot flashes and fevers persisted each evening. So on a weekend in mid-March, we drove up to the mountains and skied again. I fared much better on the slopes this time, able to get in a few ski runs before my body cramped up again. But at least I felt it was a little progress. Somehow, during the course of the day, I tweaked a pectoral muscle. I had noticed some soreness and tenderness in the muscle below my right clavicle. We were staying in a condo at the ski resort, and that night, I put a heating pad on the muscle and slept with it. In the morning, I woke up and the muscle had swollen to the size of half a grapefruit. Chris took one look at it and said it didn't look right at all. The tenderness went all the way to my right armpit, and I was thinking I had some weird, painful growth.

Back to the doctor I went to have this area examined. During our meeting, I told her the fatigue, night sweats, and evening fevers continued, and I wasn't sleeping. She examined the area that was swollen and said I pulled a muscle. We determined it was from dragging my ski pole behind me. (I tend to ski fast, and the very bad habit of dragging my pole slows me down.) I had overworked the muscle. I asked her about the tenderness in my armpit, and she showed me how this particular muscle attaches in the armpit. *Okay, no tumor, no swollen lymph node,* I thought. She somewhat scolded me and said, "Look, I know you want to get out and be active, but you really need to give your body rest—you have mono. Give your body a chance to heal." She prescribed me Vicodin for the muscle pain and Valium as a sleep aid.

Two weeks later, I was in her office for a planned follow-up exam and more blood tests to see if the mono had gone away. I was still having all the same symptoms, although the Valium did help me sleep better. In the interim, I continued to do research on my symptoms and came across chronic fatigue syndrome. The description I read of this illness fit everything I was feeling: in particular, the way my muscles behaved after physical exertion was described to a T. While no cure exists for this syndrome, several hundred thousand people live with the disorder. Could this possibly be the answer I was looking for?

I had also sought the care of an acupuncturist, recommended to me by my sister. After I'd seen him for two weeks with only a slight improvement, he talked to me about *candida albicans.* Everyone has candida, or yeast, in their bodies. For some people, this yeast overgrows in the intestines. It can make you chronically sick and produce the very symptoms I was experiencing. I took a couple of different written assessment tests for this condition (there is no existing medical test that shows yeast overgrowth) and scored high. Perhaps this was the answer. The treatment for candida overgrowth is a detoxification program that gently cleanses the digestive tract and kills the bad bacteria and yeast, while promoting growth of good yeast. I spent a couple of hours researching this on the Internet and browsed a couple of books at the bookstore, and agreed with my acupuncturist that this could be what I was suffering from.

I told my family doctor on my follow-up visit what I was able to find out relating to my symptoms, and that I was intending to go on a candida detox program. She thought that would be okay, but added, "I am concerned about your weight loss and starting this type of program, which is very restrictive on what you can eat." She told me to proceed with caution and to see her again if any of my symptoms worsened. A few days later, I checked on the results from the latest round of blood tests and my blood counts were back to normal—the mono was gone.

It was now April 2008, and still feeling much fatigue and exhaustion, even with the mono cleared, I embarked on a twelve-week candida detoxification program and continued to see my acupuncturist weekly. The diet eliminated all sugars, refined foods, processed foods, dairy, wine, and cheese. What? No wine and cheese? These were practically staples in my diet. I also drank a detoxification mix of bentonite, caporyl oil, and psyllium seed twice daily to cleanse and kill the bad bacteria. In addition, I took probiotics to restore the good bacteria, and after a couple of weeks, I started to feel marginal improvement. I was beginning to add some social activity to my calendar when I could.

It was May 2008 when I hit a wall with the detox regimen, feeling no improvement for several days, and some of the same symptoms that had subsided somewhat were starting to magnify again. By this point, most of 2008 had been marked with dealing with my ill health, having only enough energy to work a full week and then spend the weekend recovering to start the work week all over again. Both Chris and I were getting pretty frustrated with my health issues not improving. We started talking about the possibility of my taking a medical leave of absence from work so I could focus 100 percent of my time on finding answers to and improving my health. I couldn't live like this any longer. For two consecutive weeks in May, I had a headache daily, and my neck and back muscles, which had some improvement from the few physical therapy sessions, were starting to knot up badly again. I would take Excedrin Migraine every day to treat my headaches, but I realized I couldn't rely on this forever. I thought maybe it was time to get my eyes checked and made an appointment. Turns out I needed progressive lenses (trifocals), and I ordered a pair of new glasses. I thought that would help diminish my headaches.

Then, I went on a business trip the week before Memorial Day. The trip was scheduled for three days, but I ended up cutting it short and coming back early. My body crashed—I couldn't take running through the airport, toting my luggage and briefcase. I was completely exhausted and overcome with a horribly painful migraine. I called my acupuncturist and explained to him what was going on. I was seven weeks into a twelve-week detox program and not feeling better. "Shouldn't I be getting better?" I asked him. He told me I needed to be patient. Not exactly the words I wanted to hear. I had been dealing with feeling like crap for months. By this time, I had been starving myself for seven weeks, and my weight was now down thirty pounds since November. (I am only five feet, one inch tall and have a small frame, so thirty pounds is a lot of weight.) After I got off the phone with the acupuncturist, I decided I was through with him and the candida detox diet. I was going back to eating whatever I wanted (provided I had the appetite). I also made another appointment with my family doctor that Friday before Memorial Day.

On May 24, 2008, I met with my family doctor in her office for what would turn out to be the last time. It had been two months since my last visit, and she immediately was concerned about my weight loss—more than twenty pounds since I first started seeing her at the beginning of the year. I reported to her what I'd been doing over the past two months for my health, what happened on my business trip, the symptoms I continued to have: chronic fatigue, migraines, night sweats (they had subsided somewhat, possibly due to the acupuncture), etc. I told her I needed to find out what was going on, that I couldn't live like this anymore, and I needed her help with exploring a medical leave of absence. At this point, I just broke down and cried, feeling complete and utter helplessness at having to admit that I could not work and try to figure out what was wrong with me at the same time—I just didn't have the energy for it. She empathized, told me she would work with me on a leave of absence, and explained what was required was to start a health care program with her that would include physical and mental care. She revisited, again, my anxiety. We talked about my coping level, and she asked if I was ready to take a look again at depression medication. At that point, she finally was able to break me of my resistance to a depression diagnosis. After all, my coping skills were at zero, and so I gave in and said yes, give me anything. She told me the antidepressant she would recommend was not addicting; it was only to get my coping skills to a level playing field so I could address my real health concerns. She also prescribed more physical therapy and referred me to a psychologist. She drew more blood, but this time ordered only blood work to test for thyroid level, lupus, and inflammation. I left her office feeling better that I was on some sort of plan.

The following Tuesday, my doctor called me with the results. She sounded surprised: My thyroid was normal, but I tested high for lupus and inflammation. "It doesn't mean lupus is conclusive," she said. "It means I need to refer you to a specialist, a rheumatologist, to take more tests to determine what's going on." *Okay, finally some progress*, I thought. I set an appointment with the referral but couldn't get in to see him for three weeks. I was still determined to take a medical leave of absence soon, but Chris and I first had a vacation scheduled with his parents.

We flew to his hometown in Alabama and then drove several hours with his parents to the panhandle of Florida to celebrate their fortieth wedding anniversary. I was tired during the trip but felt good enough to enjoy the beach and the company. Chris and I returned a week later, on Wednesday, June 4, and I was back at work on Thursday and Friday—for the last time. My body was starting to crash again. *That's it*, I decided, and I called my family doctor and scheduled an appointment with her on Monday to proceed with the medical-leave paperwork. My plan was to take a couple of days to tidy up loose ends and prepare people at work for my leave of absence, which would begin the following Wednesday. But little did I know what lay ahead for me that weekend.

It was Sunday, June 8. I woke up feeling very lethargic and weaker than my normal state of weakness. I got up to make breakfast but could barely stand over the stove. I kept leaning on the kitchen counter, resting my head in my hands. Additionally, some numbness I had been feeling on the left side of my chin for several days had now spread to the right side of my chin. None of this was good, and I knew it. By early afternoon, I called my doctor's answering service, as I was concerned that maybe these issues should be looked at today, rather than waiting to see her on Monday. She wasn't on call, but another doctor from her office called me back. I explained to him what was happening, but since he didn't know anything about my history, it was difficult for him to determine if this was an emergency. He told me if I felt as if I needed to be seen that day that I should go to the emergency room. He wasn't much help. Chris was beside himself, insisting that I get checked out, and after a couple more hours, he convinced me. I told him if we went to the emergency room, they would surely admit me. I remember my mom having to go to the emergency room a couple of years earlier complaining of numbness in her face, and generally speaking, that means an overnight stay until they can figure it out. Chris packed us an overnight bag in anticipation.

Once I was in a room at the ER at Sky Ridge Medical Center, I had to explain my history and story at least five times to different medical aides, nurses, and finally the ER doctor. One of the nurses who examined me looked at my tongue and my gums and asked me if I was anemic. I told her I wasn't aware if I was or not. Because of the numbness in my face, the ER doctor ordered a CT scan of the head, but he told me since

I was already on a path with my current family doctor and meeting with a rheumatologist soon, he didn't want to subject me to a battery of blood tests. He was ready to send me home if the CT scan came back normal. He walked out of my room and I heard him talk with the nurse, who insisted that he not let me leave without first checking me for anemia. He acquiesced and ordered blood tests. Within fifteen minutes, he was back in my room with the results.

"This is an instance where it's best the doctor listen to his nurse. Your blood count is dangerously low. You have half the amount you should have. We're going to transfuse you with two units of blood, and we need to do it immediately." He also said he had talked to the hospital's admitting doctor as he determined that I would need to get admitted "based on the fact that it will take a while for the blood transfusion, and we also need time to find why you're losing blood."

Over the next hour in the ER, I was examined to determine if I was bleeding internally. Once that was ruled out, I was sent to radiology for a CT scan of my head. Next was a chest x-ray. Back in my room, the doctor told me the results for the CT head scan came back negative, while the chest x-ray showed an area of congestion around my lungs. He ordered a chest CT scan, and I was wheeled off to radiology again. Once back in my room, I was beginning to receive my first unit of blood, when the ER doctor walked in with the results of the chest CT scan. It was somewhat disconcerting to him that two hours earlier he almost sent me home, but because of a nurse's keen awareness and insistence, he was now in my room telling me the following in a slow, deliberate, and serious tone: "The chest CT scan indicates abnormalities in all of your chest lymph nodes. We usually see this type of picture in patients who have lymphoma. I am so sorry to have to deliver this kind of news. You need to know that lymphoma is very treatable, and you will receive the best care possible." He explained that lymphoma is a blood disease and a hematologist would come by my hospital room on Monday to determine the next steps. Finally, some preliminary answers. But the news was shocking to me and Chris.

I got more answers about my condition in those two hours at the emergency room than I had in eight months of searching and living with the frustration of poor health. Although the eventual diagnosis was scary to face, the prognosis was very good. Hodgkin's lymphoma nodular sclerosis, stage IV-B, even in the latest stage of the disease, is still very treatable. My life has been forever altered because of this disease. I am ready to face the challenges head-on and am determined to be cancer-free.

A Full-Time Job

I had a terrific weekend. Prudy must have finally kicked in and boosted my red blood cell count, as I had more energy Saturday and Sunday. Today, however, I'm a little off. I'm not sure why, except that I ran an errand earlier today and I guess these little outings really kick my butt.

I went back to Linda's Boutique to meet with Mary. She had a couple other wig colors for me to try out, and one was almost a perfect match to my current hair color. I went ahead and purchased a rug. She fitted the piece onto my head and then removed it to sew the crown area to adjust the cap to the shape of my head. Apparently, the back of my head is flat, "not rounded like most people," she quipped. She slipped the wig back on my head, and it was nice and snug. Then she cut off the wig's length into a style close to the bob I've been recently sporting. It's cute and looks like my real hair. And just in time. I have been shedding and pulling out clumps of hair all weekend; it is now more than half gone. My hair has still been shedding proportionally, so I still have a style to it, although I expect this thinner bob version to be gone in a matter of days. I may just cut it short to the scalp. Mary advised against shaving my head bald because an even stubble creates an even pressure all over the scalp, which is already tender from the trauma of chemo and hair loss.

The wig fitting took two and a half hours. Beating cancer is a full-time job. Chris and I then went to lunch down the street at a small restaurant, Cozy Cottage, which Mary had recommended. What a great place. It only had five tables in the joint, and they serve breakfast all day. I ordered lunch, even though anyone who knows me knows that I love, love breakfast. Since I had already had breakfast, I didn't want to pour more cholesterol or sugar in my body. My first outing with my fake hair, and no one knew the difference.

When we arrived home, the cleaning ladies we recently hired were finishing their house chores. I wondered what they thought about all the hair they were mopping and vacuuming up. My brother came over to hang out with me, and then my body sort of crashed and needed some sleep. I'm very headachy and worn out. I hope my blood counts are good enough to start chemo tomorrow. I am actually anxious to start cycle two so I can get past it. Completing each cycle is like a mini-goal, and I look forward to marking a big fat X through my appointment calendar showing completion of each one. That means I am on my way to kicking this cancer's ass. I want my life back.

CYCLE TWO

Finding Comforts

Heavenly Instruments

Cycle two has begun, and I am more tired than I have felt in this whole process. Today has me down, but not out. Prudy didn't do enough for me and I had to get another shot, this time a higher dosage. The fatigue is from a low count of red blood cells. Red blood cells carry oxygen throughout your body, and having a low count has the effect of making me feel like I've been flattened by a Mack truck. Brother Rick was with me throughout my six-hour ordeal in the doctor's office today. It was nice to have him there and spend time together.

When we got home this afternoon, I slept for a while. When I awoke, Rick was on my computer on YouTube, watching videos of various musical artists. For those who don't know, Rick has amazing musical talents. He sings, composes, and is self-taught on the piano. He wrote a song for Chris and me and performed it at our wedding reception two and a half years ago. He rocks. So, we're sitting there and he pulls up a video of this fourteen-year-old phenom from the Philippines. I was literally blown away by this young girl's singing voice. This petite, pubescent child had mastered soulfulness as she sang Whitney Houston songs with the depth of emotions only mature broken-hearted adults know. I couldn't help but be totally moved by this incredible talent, and listening to her lifted my spirits and my energy level as I watched in awe. What an inspiration.

Chris had heard us from the room across the hall, so not to be outdone, he walked over and told us to look up a five-year-old blind pianist he had seen featured in an online article a couple of days ago. We looked her up on YouTube as well. Here was yet another incredibly talented, adorable little girl from South Korea, playing Mozart! She had to sit on someone's lap just to reach the keys, which she could only feel and not see. Her precious little hands and fingers attacked the piano with such passion far beyond her years I couldn't help but be affected in such a glorious way, watching her.

What gifts these are to me, given at a time when I am feeling pretty low. The beauty in it is so incomprehensible, it is perfection. I cannot help but believe in a higher power, forces of the universe, God—take your pick—sending me messages right when I need them, showing me life and love and the purity of the human heart and soul, the absolute magnificence of being. I am so full of hope, of joy, of love. This moment wasn't mine alone, I got to share it with my brother and my husband. The universe is using my family, my friends as instruments to my healing, and I am eternally grateful and more determined than ever to reclaim my health.

The Paradox of Cancer

A much better day today—it's like night and day. I had lots of energy, despite my three-hour chemo appointment turning into a five-hour visit. I had another allergic reaction to one of the chemo drugs, which slowed the treatment process today. My doctor physically checked my neck and armpit lymph nodes and said they are smaller! Great news today. Six to eight cycles of this? Yeah, right. My personal goal is four, and when I told him that, he looked sideways at me, eyes narrowed—not so fast, girlfriend, we want this done right. As do I.

My sister and brother were both with me, giving Chris some much-needed relief to finish wrapping things up at his current job (at the company where I am still employed but on short-term disability) before he starts his new one on Monday.

Cancer presents an interesting paradox: it is a challenging illness, yet it brings so many blessings to your life. One of the blessings for me has been reconnecting, renewing a wonderful relationship with my sister Jeanette. We have gone on more than a quarter century of our adult lives feeling close but not really being intimately involved with each other's lives. During the beginning of this journey of mine, from my days in the hospital to now, she has been surprised to find out the deep network of friends and support that I have. Of course she knew I had friends, but in living our lives so differently, she didn't know any of them, and thus, she didn't really know this side of me. And while we have spent hundreds of days and thousands of hours together on her kids' birthdays and all the family holidays, there were usually so many people around we didn't really have time (or sadly, made no effort to find the time) to spend one-on-one together, although our love for each other was always there. At times, this lack of involvement in each other's lives has caused confusion, conflict, and sometimes heartache in not truly knowing each other intimately.

Our paths were so different. Jeanette was a teenage mother of two girls before she met her husband and married at age twenty-two. She has five children, from ages thirteen to twenty-seven. And she is the proud grandmother of a beautiful sixteen-month-old girl. She has been a full-time working mother the entire time, managing the office and operations of a successful dental business, and she has been a good wife, despite some bumps in the road that often come when people marry so young. Jeanette is forty-five now, and it is amazing what she has accomplished in that quarter century of adulthood. I have always marveled at her strength and admired her—probably too much from afar.

I took a different path, one filled with many years living a single life, chasing a career, chasing men, and them chasing me (chasing, chasing, chasing). After years of the chase, I was happily accepting the fate of no-such-thing-as-a-soulmate-at-least-for-me, and that's literally right when love knocked me off my feet. At age forty, I married my soulmate. No kids, and probably none in the future. (This illness is putting an exclamation point on that notion.) I have lived vicariously through my sister's life, watching her raise such beautiful children. And as a doting, loving aunt, I thank her for them. Since the age of sixteen, I have been very blessed to have grown up with children in my life because of her.

Now our paths are crossing in this paradox of challenge and blessing. This quarter century later, I am getting to know my sister as a true friend, a best friend. And she is equally enjoying getting to know her baby sister as a true friend, a best friend. The bond and love of sisterhood is deepening, and I look forward to the next twenty-five years and beyond. And so I proclaim here tonight, my UBFF, Ultimate Best Friend Forever, my sister, Jeanette.

* * *

Night and day again—this time, it's night. I am beat. Day three of chemo has knocked it out of me. Whew. Low blood count, disappointing, but tomorrow I'll go in for a couple units of blood. Nothing perks you up like a pint or two of hemoglobin. The Procrit is working to some extent, but the chemo drugs break you down at the same time. It is a delicate balancing act. I'm learning so much.

My sister has been by my side at the doctor's office and is staying a little afterwards while I rest at home. It is so comforting to have her here. She returns tomorrow to cook me breakfast. This morning was yummy blueberry pancakes, and tomorrow it will be my favorite veggie omelets before I get the transfusion.

Brother Rick and Ron are on their way over to bring me some chicken cacciatore. Again, yum! They will need to dine with me in the upstairs retreat, as I am too tired to sit around the dinner table tonight. Need to preserve my energy. I received many phone calls today; I couldn't get to or return all of them. I'll try to return calls after I get the juice of life. Signing off for now.

The Comfort of Mac-n-Cheese

Have you ever had one of those perfect days? That's how I would describe today. In spite of the challenges I am facing and the fact that I am so blurry-eyed I can barely see or concentrate too long (having just taken another Benadryl), I feel so compelled to write about it.

It started out with my sister cooking the veggie omelet this morning. Then, dear friends of Chris's stopped by to see me before I left for my blood transfusion. Their lives have been turned upside down because of a career move (a good one), which has them moving to Chicago with their four children *tomorrow*, a development that has happened in about two weeks. They knew I had a scheduled appointment but drove the forty miles from the north side of town anyway to personally wish me well before embarking on their new lives. It was only a ten-minute visit, but it meant the world to me.

Off to Sky Ridge I went, and the infusion of blood gave me another reaction. With all that my body is going through ingesting drugs via mouth or IV, it is trying to process so much, and at times, it's overloaded. The result is an allergic reaction. My body rebels, releasing histamines that cause my skin to blotch with red patches and my breath to labor. The nurses counteract these outbreaks with Benadryl and lots of fluid, but it continues to be a balancing act. My sister again by my side, as we work through our therapy sessions together—how I enjoy the time! My brother also came by, and the three of us reminisced about our childhood and how our lives have been so impacted by family, each other.

Then home again, to see my wonderful husband, who has been transitioning to his new job, one that will be challenging but I am confident most rewarding. My sister prepared a dinner that was divine— and at my request, homemade mac-n-cheese with chicken; her first attempt at a new recipe that knocked everyone's socks off.

My beautiful niece and her husband traveled many miles with their adorable sixteen-month-old daughter, whom I haven't seen since this whole journey of mine began, to dine with us this evening. And there on my wood floors was this wondrous child playing, laughing, and making my spirit soar. I was soooo tired, but I could not tear myself away from this perfection of a day.

And earlier, as I watched my niece's husband help my sister in the kitchen, we got a chance to catch up. His great-uncle and childhood father figure is in hospice care, facing death from melanoma that has metastasized. It is a matter of time, he says. Despite this heavy burden, my nephew-in-law is handling it with such courage, and there he stood in my kitchen shredding cheese and roast chicken, helping my sister cook that amazing meal—all to make me feel better.

Everything I see, everything I taste, I am drinking it up like the earth, which soaked in the drenching rain that passed over our house in a burst of energy right before dinner. I am collecting every wonderfully tender moment, every heartfelt comment and kind gesture, basically all of life unfolding underneath me, around me, and putting them in my bucket of hope, dreams, and the future. I am drawing strength from it all, and it will hold me up and sustain me throughout this process. My life is forever changed.

Tuning In

This has been a much better weekend energywise, although Friday evening, after my perfect day and dinner, was a little rough. I ended up calling my doctor's answering service around 9:00 PM. When you notice that your husband keeps staring at you with a look of concern as he periodically pulls your shirt aside and touches the redness on your neck and chest, coupled with the fact that you feel your own breath getting more and more labored … well, it makes you think, is something wrong?

Each time I get a blood infusion, I am given a list of certain symptoms to watch out for (such as the ones I was experiencing), along with the instruction to call my doctor if any of these occur accompanied by a sudden onset of anxiety; these may indicate an emergency situation. Your brain plays tricks on you, though, and like I said, when your husband is looking at you with concern, the anxiety level tends to peak. So it was best I called.

The doctor on call was one of the other oncologists in the practice, and she talked me through what I was feeling in a very calming and comforting fashion. I told her I had a reaction earlier that day to the blood transfusion, and she determined that my body was still trying to process all that was happening to it, even hours after the infusion. She could tell that I wasn't too labored in my breathing and stepped me through what would happen if I did decide to go to the emergency room having just gone through a blood transfusion that day. Simply put, they would give me saline solution, steroids, just some basic help for my body to process what was going on. That was a relief. At least my heart wasn't going to stop or explode and my body wasn't rejecting the blood. And knowing that this was nothing serious, my husband and I were able to relax. I took another Benadryl and went to bed.

I have a very good medical team; they seem to be one of the best. Whenever I mention the name of the practice or any of the doctors to others in the medical field, the response is very positive and an affirmation of *Yes, they are the best in what they do*. It's very comforting. My doctor has incredible confidence in the body's ability to heal, and he exudes that confidence to me. This week, while the nurses seemed concerned that my blood counts were teetering on being potentially too low to start chemo, he simply said, "Go ahead with the treatment. Let's see how she does." And when my hemoglobin count hit that number that they don't like it to go below, he calmly ordered me to get blood. I have asked him about other things I can do with my body to aid in its recovery, such as a detox for my liver, even coffee enemas or hydrocolonics. His belief in the human body to heal itself even with chemo is strong, so he doesn't tell me *not* to do these things, he just says, "If you want to put yourself through these regimens, go for it." I will likely add other natural ways to help my body process, despite his clinical view. But I very much understand and appreciate how he and the medicine are treating and, in a way, manipulating my body to health. I take a host of oral prescription drugs and over-the-counter medicine now, and I am very careful with timing these drugs throughout the day to give my liver and body a break. I am not one to pop all the pills once in the morning and be done with it—too hard on the body, I think. I am becoming more aware and tuned in to what my body needs through this process and which over-the-counter medicine to take to offset side effects from the chemo and steroids. I know when to rest. I am listening.

Saturday was a better day for energy, and another one filled to near perfection. A good friend came over to cook me and Chris breakfast. It was quite de-lish! And later that morning, I received a phone call from my aunts, uncles, and cousins at the reunion that we were not able to attend. One by one, they each gave me well-wishes and love and told me they missed having me and all the Colorado gang with them this year. It was like I was there—I could see each of their faces and feel their love and hugs. One of my uncles made my heart skip a beat, his voice sounded so much like my father's.

In the afternoon, Chris talked me into going to a movie. We went to see *Mamma Mia!* and loved it! What a sight we must have been. It was a hot summer day, but even so, I covered up all exposed skin to protect it from the sun (as instructed by the nurses because the chemo and steroids make the skin very sensitive to sunlight and sunburning). I also don't walk very fast these days, fatigued by the full-time battle. So, there I was on Chris's arm, walking slowly, sporting a wide-brimmed sunhat and big, dark sunglasses, long-sleeved shirt, and pants. People probably thought what a nice young man he was taking his mother to the movies!

In the bathroom after the movie, I noticed the looks of curiosity from some of the theater patrons, but for the most part, the expressions were of kindness and empathy, and I could tell they wondered what might be wrong with me. I didn't mind; I know it's the same way I have reacted whenever I've seen a person who appeared somewhat challenged—never with pity, but compassion. And also I didn't mind because I was out on an afternoon date with my husband and thoroughly enjoyed the movie.

Back at home, we were taking a little catnap, when one of my nieces stopped by for a visit. I haven't seen her since my stay in the hospital six weeks ago; she hadn't been over with her mom, my sister, during one of the many Saturday family gatherings at my house. Turns out she had stayed away trying to process what was going on with her Auntie Barbie, waiting to spend some time with me when she was ready. She hadn't really kept up-to-date on my journaling, she said when I asked her; some things are too close. But having her spend those few hours with me and Chris that day was like watching a flower blossom in a young, beautiful girl, full of such insight and wisdom for her age. At twenty-one, she has this depth in her soul that I only had glimpses of when I was that age. On occasion, I would get lost in her gorgeous, liquid-green eyes that felt like they were drinking in my tiredness and gently caressing my weary body. She and Chris connected on a lot of issues, and it was wonderful to watch their exchange. We talked about the abstract, the gift and beauty of life. I smiled as I thought to myself, *She is going to heal many people in her lifetime.*

Transitions

There are benefits to being hairless. Showers are much shorter. My previous thick head of hair used to add a good thirty minutes to my morning routine if I washed, conditioned, and combed in the shower, towel dried and then conditioned and combed again (my long, coarse hair needed dual conditioning action), dried, straightened, and styled. Geez, writing about it is exhausting. I have found thirty minutes in my day. Although I must admit, I am anxious to give them back for some gorgeous locks. And shaving? No need. Hair isn't there, and it ain't growing *anywhere*. Which certainly cuts down on the expense of not only haircuts but lip, eyebrow, and yes, bikini waxing. A good thing, since those dollars can now be spent on scarves, wigs, and hats. Life has an uncanny way of balancing itself out.

And let's talk food, because I cannot seem to get enough of it lately. I am a pig (in the nicest way, of course). I am eating four to five times a day; one day, I ate seven times. I am talking full meals here. Okay, not *every* meal is full, but at least three are, with an additional two to three small meals—*a day*! But considering I had no appetite for several months, this is a small miracle. And, as the balance of life promises, that means my waistline will also share in that small miracle, and eventually in a big way. The alternative to this is I could have no appetite, lots of nausea, and continued weight loss. So, count me as lucky—at least, that is what my medical team says, as they prefer to see healthy appetites and weight gain. Even the gas pain doesn't deter me. These changes are all thanks to my little friend, prednisone. That is one steroid *on* steroids.

I have had a string of three good days of energy and am shooting for four tomorrow. Just about enough energy to resume walking in the mornings. I even baked cookies today. Can you say *Martha Stewart?* Even my husband was amazed at my energy. I took my last oral chemo drug today, and tomorrow it's back to the doctor's office for day eight of IV, the short day. They'll also draw blood, and I expect good results. I wonder if I'll get a shot of Prudy tomorrow. I may not need the gerbil ovaries. But I'm pretty sure I'll get Nesta, as is usual on day nine. E. coli—yay.

Chris started his new job today. We got a large package delivered from FedEx. You could have fit a body in that box. Inside was an all-in-one fax, printer, scanner, and goodness knows what else it can do. He spent the day setting up his office and making all his initial contacts. Already, he has to travel this week and probably a night or two next week. It is amazing to think what he has gone through the past several weeks, dealing with his ill wife, doing his best to make my life manageable, workable, and getting me healthy, all while transitioning jobs. He is the best husband in the world.

A Question of Worth

Another great day feeling good. Good, of course, is relative. Good means "okay to be on chemotherapy" good, and managing just fine. Today, my red blood cell count showed a boost, but the white blood cell count is *dangerously* low. The doctors and nurses use that word—*dangerously*—to describe a white blood cell count at one or below. (Specifically, it means I have 1,000 or fewer white cells per cubic millimeter of blood.) I'm not sure of its relevancy either. *Dangerously* low for a normal healthy person? (A normal healthy range is between 4.1 and 11 or 4,100 and 11,000 cells.) Or just for me? In any event, the nurse practitioner said I could have been hospitalized and doped up with antibiotics, that's how *dangerously* low I am, but it must not be that dangerous, as my doctor let me go home after today's chemo treatment.

Stay home, away from sick people, don't eat raw fruits and vegetables. Of course, I had a big bowl of infection-potential blueberries and strawberries before I went in for treatment this morning. That's okay, the nurse said. *Really?* You just told me to avoid the stuff. Watch for a temperature spike. Anything over 100.5, call the doctor. But, then again, your temperature may not rise because you have zippo white blood cells anyway, which is what you need to raise a temperature if you get an infection. So instead, you need to be aware of chills only and no fever. Oy! And while you're at it, that incredible gas pain would surely go away if you would just stop pigging out. And it probably would help with the bowel movement if you stopped eating so much.

Pigging out seems to be my choice, but isn't that the prednisone affecting me? Can I control the steroid-induced appetite—*do I want to?* The scales are tipping, almost ten pounds in one month. All around my little midsection. Mostly bloated, some water retention, the rest good ol' fat cells. Do I care? I'm not sure yet—the food tastes too good. Plus, it's a little comforting how the food makes me feel, particularly since other things are truly inconvenient, like my chemo-drip nose and nosebleeds, and dry skin and cracking fingernail beds, and oh yeah, the hair loss, gas pain, and extreme fatigue. And, oh, by the way, I have stage IV cancer. Screw it, I am eating.

Big bro Rick kept me company today during treatment. We talked a lot about books and writing. Clearly, writing is in my future in some way, shape, or form. To be able to have a vision, a passion, a creative outlet, which this writing and posting in my journal is providing me, is so freeing and makes my heart sing. I am genuinely, seriously, deliriously happy. What craziness is that, given how sick I am? The *absurdity* of it all. Why am I okay with being kicked on my butt with this cancer, but so willing to go through the crappiness of it all to discover this incredible, happy spirit of mine? Better yet, why did this need to happen in order for me to find it? I thought I was already a pretty positive, upbeat, friendly, happy, decent human being. I had already found true love and a great husband, was surrounded by an amazing family and fabulous friends, and had a good, successful career. Why am I being given this chance (gift? blessing?) to go even deeper into myself, to be even happier? *Why?* And why am I even questioning why? What do I do with this gift? Whom do I help? These questions keep swirling around my mind, sometimes like a cyclone with no direction, other times like a warm ocean breeze with full knowing. It is the most bizarre thing to be in my chemo-hazed brain right now.

What is most absurd is that I am questioning my own happiness, or rather whether I *deserve* to be happy. Now that is crazy, as I would shout from the highest mountaintops that surely everyone deserves happiness. I would slay dragons in order that my best of friends and all my family be able to stake their claim on a right to be happy. Why on earth am I questioning my own worthiness? Catholic guilt? No. Whenever I feel really good, almost invincible, like things have come to me somewhat easily in waves of good luck and blessings, I hear this nagging voice behind me, *Who do you think you are, being so happy? Do you deserve to be here? How* audacious *of you.* Now, I will tell you that this is pretty deep stuff; it is fucked up, really, and at the heart of my psyche—this questioning of worthiness has been with me my entire life. But I think I know the demons that afflict my mind. And of course, we only have our parents to blame, right? Okay, that's not a fair assessment, but typically whenever we delve this deep into our souls, generally speaking, we examine what happened in our childhood. And I do recall childhood memories of being told I wasn't worthy—*by my own mother.* Now, before anyone jumps on my mom, I will surely kick your ass, so don't go there.

This is a story of my mom, how much I am not like her, and how much I am like her. Will she read this? I don't know. She doesn't like to read. I remember once I gave her a book by Priscilla Presley, *Elvis and Me*—I think that was the title. If you know my mother, she is the biggest Elvis Presley fan. Next to my father, Elvis is the man she idolized, worshipped, and loved—of course, she and millions of other frenzied, hip-glaring, adoring fans. And you would think by the way she plays his music still today that she might have left my dad were Mr. Presley ever to wink in her direction. So, giving her this book about what it was actually like to be married to Elvis, live with him, love him, you would think that was a good gift, right? Wrong. First of all, Mom watches and observes. Reading is not her thing. Secondly, she was in love with Elvis, so why on earth would she care what Priscilla thought or how she loved and lived with him? Mom had her own fantasies and could not have given a hoot about Priscilla Presley. I missed the boat completely. There is so much I had to and still need to learn about my mom. And now, through this illness, this phase of my life, I am starting to get it.

My mother is a simple, take-no-prisoners, strong woman at the age of seventy-one. She will tell you exactly what is on her mind; there is no editing or pre-thought or tact. It is out there. Sometimes it's funny, but oftentimes, what spills off those tightly pursed but sweet lips is hypercritical and painful. Over the years, I have taught myself to translate these zings and zaps and stand them straight on their tops, then spin them 180 degrees to a compliment. Doing this has made me able to better communicate with Mom; I can look at her in a softer light. For example, if I came back from a relaxing vacation on a tropical beach, sporting a gorgeous, golden tan, my mother would say something like, "Barbara, why are you getting *so* much sun? Your skin is *too dark*, it is *so ugly!*" Without hesitation, I would gather these words in my head and translate them to something like, *Barbara, I'm* so happy *to see you so refreshed and relaxed from your vacation. Did you have a good time? Now, I am concerned about too much sun exposure you may be getting, but you look radiant and beautiful.* Rather than furrowing my brow and scowling back at her with some smart-ass retort to her actual words, I would reply to the translated, more complimentary version in my head and say, "Thanks for your concern about my skin, Mom. But I am careful in the sun, and I do like my tan."

I remember the day I made this conscious decision to view my mother differently than I had growing up as a child and teenager. I was twenty-one and talking to my then-roommate about my mother's life and how she met my dad in the Philippines. She was a twenty-two-year-old single mother of two children—boys, ages four and eighteen months—when she met my father at the air force officer's club. Mom was part of a group of young women—dance escorts—who were brought to the officer's club to dance with the young servicemen. This was fifty years ago. It was a time of innocence and respectfulness—nothing like the wild or lewd stories you hear about today on the Internet or cable news regarding dance clubs or dancing girls catering to our boys overseas. We (society) are so desensitized and decades away from that simple life of when two people like my parents met and fell in love. When I had finished telling my mom's story of how she arrived here in America, my roommate said to me, "Your mother sounds like an amazing person." Up until that point, *amazing* was not a word I used to describe my mother. And I didn't think her story was that remarkable. I paused and in that moment began to appreciate my mother's history. And that's when I changed from simply regurgitating my mother's tale to actually relating to it—and to her.

They were an inseparable couple from day one, Mom and Dad (kind of like me and Chris). At the time, Mom lived away from her hometown, making her way in the world, trying to find a better place for those boys. The Philippines is an impoverished country, with a wide gap between those with means and those without. Her childhood days growing up in a small village were about survival, fishing off the deep waters for food to supply and nourish her big extended family. And the fishing stories she would talk about! In the early mornings and evenings, they would get in their small, wooden boats and row far off the shores, where Mom and the other good swimmers would jump off the boat into the deep ocean and literally grab fish. "Were there sharks?" I would ask. "Well, yes, we knew they were out there, but you had to eat," she would tell me. The boats would circle around the children (yes, they were children) in the water gathering the day's meals, and the men on the boats would be on the lookout. The children were agile and small, which made it easy for the men to scoop up their bodies from the water should any dangers lurk nearby. They lived with family members in one- and two-room huts, without running water. She was poor, and she knew it. But this was her life.

She was seventeen when she was raped. Such strong words. I don't think that's how my mother described the event when she told me and my sister this story when I was ten or so. I don't recall my exact age, but I know I was young and we were especially curious about her eldest, Danny—the one she left behind. We knew she had two sons born in her homeland, and one, Alan, had grown up with us in America. In fact, it was around this same time that we learned that Alan was not Dad's biological son, as we had believed for years. We had assumed Alan was Dad's. Why else did they bring Alan and leave Danny behind? Our young minds were bursting with questions and demanding explanations. Alan was a toddler, she explained, and he knew Dad as his only father. "Danny was six and had been living with my mother most of his life," she said. So Mom left him there to be raised by her mother. While Danny was the result of an unwelcome and violent act, you would never know it from the way my mother talked of him. How proud she was of this boy—the love that beamed across her face as she spoke of him to me and my siblings. My mother never knew her assailant, or at least that is what I remember from her story.

Fast-forward a few years to Mom and Dad's story. When they met, Mom was a single mother raising a baby alone, and Danny was rooting his life with his maternal grandmother. After a two-year romance and courtship, when Dad's tour was up and he was heading back to the United States with his new bride, they made what must have been a heart-wrenching decision on Mom's part to leave behind her eldest child. They brought Alan back to America with them. This is the first time in my journal that I have mentioned I have two half brothers, but I do. (Danny, unfortunately, is now deceased—a story for another time. Alan has led a very difficult and challenged life and resides with my mom—also a story for another time.)

A new life was waiting in the United States of America. My father came from a nurturing, loving, grounded-in-religion family who welcomed Benny, as she was so affectionately nicknamed, short for her given name, Benita. Benita, meaning beautiful. The family also took to Alan, a cute, precocious, and curious young toddler. Within a couple of years, Mom and Dad welcomed their first child into the world, followed by three more in as many years. And so our U.S. family story begins, but Mom's was still unfolding. She spoke very little English, she explains whenever she recalls those days. Dad didn't teach her too much of our language, except he said "I love you" all the time, she would tell us with a bashful grin. Mom learned from TV most of the broken, strained accent that we siblings still to this day tease her endlessly about. (But she doesn't mind being teased by us; it makes her laugh so hard, she cries. My mother's laugh is a hearty, from-the-belly, infectious laugh, and it gets my siblings and me laughing whenever we are in earshot.)

So, imagine a life in a new world, with a wonderful new husband you so deeply love but are so desperately dependent upon, in the uproarious and changing U.S. culture of the sixties. Juxtapose the feeling of love against the angst you feel at having left your own son, your family, your culture, knowing very little of the American language and way of life. Also consider how incredibly young you are, still trying to understand your place in the world. Imagine. Now pop out four more kids, one after the other, year after year, and life is getting pretty interesting. Imagine these children growing up in the new culture you have yet to understand, while you have roots and ties to a poverty these kids will, thankfully, never experience firsthand. What questions might go through your mind? What might my mother be thinking? How did this impact her life, her self-esteem, her … *worthiness?* Did she feel lucky, blessed, being rescued from a life of poverty by the man of her dreams? Did she feel great pain at what she sacrificed for this life—watching her eldest boy grow? Did she make the right decision by leaving him? *How did I do this? Do I deserve happiness?* Now, decades later, she has a daughter asking the same question of happiness deserved.

And so it comes full circle. There is much more to tell and more richness to our story, but too much detail to put here. But as I write these words, I am naked in my emotions and my thoughts, exposed. Here it is. The question is not of me asking myself if I am worthy. The question is whether I have honored my mother in her worthiness of a life worth living. She has not asked me to honor her in this way, but here again is irony and paradox. She's probably not consciously aware that this is something she needs from me. But I can ask this question of me. It is not a question of whether or not my mother sees who I am, which has been a longing of mine since I can remember—that *she* see *me*. The question is: *do I see my mother?* And, Mom, I do. *I see you.* I see the sacrifice you have made for me and my siblings. I see a life so worthy, how can I now question whether or not my life is worthy? You aren't even aware of the pain I have felt in this emptiness of questioning whether I deserve to be happy. *Was it "your" pain I have been feeling all these years?* Did you wonder whether you deserved happiness in your life? Of course you did deserve happiness and still do. And I deserve mine. You have lived a lifetime making sure I am happy. It is time I honor that, feel your pain, kiss it on the forehead, and put it to bed. I just needed to translate—take the zings and zaps, stand them straight on their tops, spin *myself* 180 degrees, and see your life as the biggest complement to mine.

Adult Supervision

Another decent day yesterday for energy level, although I started to peter out in the evening. Jeanette came over to cook dinner, with Mom and Rick, as well as my niece, visiting. Two of my BOTS (Books on the Side) girlfriends, Alex and Kristen, also stopped by. It was great to spend time with everyone around the dinner table. Mom and Rick stayed the night, with Chris out of town. It's a good thing to have coverage, or sitters, if you will. A great comfort to me, and to Chris especially, although it makes me feel like I'm a child, or maybe a dog, needing babysitting. A child or dog that's loved completely, of course.

I didn't read to my mom the post from yesterday, but I told her about it. She opened up with some new stories. My mother likes to talk about those early days; doing so keeps everything fresh and real to her. When she tells these stories, you can see her touch, taste, and feel everything like she is there again fifty years ago. I think she would like to have her story told.

As far as supervision, Mom is here this morning and will be here again tonight, along with Rick, who will come over after work. So, it's just me and Mom today until my dear friend Tami stops over to "sit" with me. Mom doesn't drive, so I am very lucky to have others around in case something happens to me, like if my infected hangnail turns gangrenous and lands me in the hospital to receive massive doses of antibiotics or, God forbid, an amputation.

Breakfast this morning with Mom was funny. We each had to take our prescription and over-the-counter drugs, so we poured out our pills on the breakfast table and proclaimed and compared which one we take and for what ailment or prevention. A true mother-daughter moment.

I have this calmness and peacefulness about me today. I'm tired but incredibly relaxed. I slept really well last night for the first time in a long time, except for some really gassy moments during the night. Charming, I know.

Chris gets back tomorrow. It sounds like his days are quite busy, and this new job will be quite the challenge, but he seems to be enjoying it so far. I miss him very much and can't wait till he gets home.

The First of Many Fevers

100.7. *Shit.*

"Rick, can you hand me the phone? I have to call the doctor." It was almost 9:00 pm last night, and I was cold. I had been battling extreme gas pain all day. I hoped the visitors I had today didn't mind the little foul rips of air my body was expunging. My good friend Tami had stayed with me most of the afternoon, and we had a good, relaxing visit. Another BOTS girlfriend, Rachel, came by with a delicious dinner. I wasn't able to eat much; the gas pain and bloatedness won the battle last night. So I was up in my retreat area lying on my chaise, and I felt a shiver. *Odd,* I thought, *better take my temperature.* It was over that gauge mark of 100.5. Rick handed me the phone and I called my doctor's answering service.

I introduced myself. "They told me to call if I spike a temperature higher than 100.5. It's at 100.7. I guess they may be concerned with my white blood count so low."

"I will page your doctor right now and patch him through." Wow, patch him right through—usually the answering service just hangs up and calls the doctor while you wait for a return call. *Is this serious?* I wondered. I waited only a minute on the line, then, "We have your doctor on the phone. Go ahead." I explained my current situation to my doctor, and that I was cold.

"Let me ask you a few questions. Do you have a sore throat or any congestion?"

"No."

"Does it burn when you urinate, or are you constipated?"

"No, I just had a bowel movement in the last hour; it was soft. I do have extreme gas pain, though. I also have this hangnail that is infected, but that's it. I am cold, but not shivering. I am tired, a little short of breath."

"Well, we do want you to call when your temperature spikes. It doesn't sound like you have any localized symptoms that are concerning. Go ahead and take two extra-strength Tylenol to get your fever down, and continue to take that every four to six hours through the night. If you feel bad in the morning, you can go in to have your blood checked at the Hampden office." I explained to him I already had a blood draw scheduled in the afternoon. "Good," he said.

Whew. I popped a couple of Tylenol and napped. Maybe that Nesta shot was finally working, because I clearly had enough white blood cells to produce a rise in temperature. An hour later, I took my temperature again. It was 101.6. *Double shit!* Rick seemed a little concerned, but I told him I'd keep checking it, the Tylenol just needed to kick in. It did in another hour, 100.3, then just thirty minutes later, 99.5. It was coming down. I broke a little sweat even, indicating the temperature had peaked and was falling. I was very tired, my gas pains had finally subsided some, and I went to bed after 11:00 pm, but set my alarm for two hours later so I could take more Tylenol.

I got up this morning after 6:00 am to eat a small breakfast with my prednisone. That is my daily routine through the fourteen days I have to take that steroid per cycle. One of the drug's side effects is insomnia, which is why I pop my sixty milligrams so early in the morning and with a side order of food to minimize stomach irritation. I then go back upstairs and nap for one to two hours before getting up again and making round two of breakfast. (Remember; breakfast is my favorite meal.) While I was napping between the two meals, my stomach continued to churn with air. The chemo and this drug are wreaking havoc on my digestive tract. I was still a little feverish and took more Tylenol. I just started sobbing. I am tired. This pain hurts. The effects of all the drugs are taking away one of my comforts—food. I don't want to give in to this and not eat.

It is now after noon and I haven't had lunch. My stomach continues to rumble with gas, and I'm hesitant to put anything in it. Rick's partner, Ron, will be here to take me to my lab appointment in an hour. I will ask the nurse what else I can do for the gas pain. And, of course, I hope my counts are good.

Mashed Potatoes and Gravy

Balance. Equilibrium. Yin and Yang. Ebb and Flow. Cause and Effect. Laws of Nature. There is just so much to be said for the simple statement "Things have a way of working themselves out."

This second cycle is literally kicking me in the pants. But as I sit here, really physically exhausted, with stomach and intestinal pain, tender hemorrhoids, sore hangnails, blurry vision, and keenly aware of the dangers of a low white blood-cell count, I am thinking about the wondrous gifts brought to me yesterday, giving me a feeling of calm and peace right now—balancing out the inconvenience of this illness.

Right before I left for my appointment for a blood draw, I received a package in the mail. The package was sent by my cousin Kathy, who just returned from the 2008 Johnson Reunion, the one the Colorado clan passed up because of this unfortunate bump in the road called cancer. Inside was a letter detailing the reunion events from last weekend, and twenty-one homemade cards of well-wishes from my uncles, aunts, and cousins. Tears streamed down my face as I opened each card—I felt the energy and rush of healing power transcend from each creator's hands to the carefully crafted construction paper, colors and crayons and glue straight to my heart, my body, my soul. These masterpieces of love contained messages of hope and joy and perfectly captured each creator's personality; each card a work of art that I will treasure forever. One of my cousins also made a T-shirt memorializing the reunion for each participant, and one of those T-shirts was also in the package with the cards. So, I have my T-shirt, I have my homemade greeting cards—I may not be in the digital pictures, *but I was there*. What an amazing gift.

And that gift arrived just in time, because the rest of my afternoon and evening, and most of today, turned out to be physically challenging. Ron took me to my blood-draw appointment Friday afternoon. I was looking forward to spending time with him. He sat with me as the lab tech checked my vitals and drew the juice of life from my veins. The results of the counts were not good (though not alarming, given what the chemo is doing to my cells). The nurse practitioner came by to give me the news of all the transfusions they just lined me up for. Starting with platelets: *You need to get that done this afternoon.* I looked at Ron, smiled, and said, "So are you ready for a little adventure?" He was game. They also ordered me to receive a blood transfusion on Saturday and Sunday.

Off to Sky Ridge Ron and I went. The nurse gave us a dramatic sendoff: *Do not get in an accident; she has virtually no clotting left in her.* Great, no white blood cells to ward off infections and not enough platelets to stop me from bleeding. Not to mention that I'm anemic, so very little oxygen is flowing through my body. Someone just put me in a plastic bubble already. (Remember that movie, *The Boy in a Plastic Bubble?* Didn't John Travolta star in that?)

The nurse at Sky Ridge who administered my blood transfusion just one week ago assisted me through the platelet transfusion Friday afternoon and the blood over the weekend. I asked her why I couldn't get all units transfused in one visit, and she said the infusion center at Sky Ridge is only open until 4:30 pm weekdays and for four hours on Saturday and Sunday. All procedures would take about eight hours. It was important that I get the platelets right away, but the blood was okay to administer over the weekend. She explained if all of this was done at once, they'd have to admit me to the hospital, which was something they wanted to avoid. I figured that the inconvenience of coming here three times and getting poked in the chest versus taking everything at once, which seems to stress my body anyway, was something I could live with. Plus no overnight hospital stay. And with Chris on an airplane on his way back home to me, unaware of this latest adventure, the last thing I wanted to do was alarm him as soon as he got off the plane with the news that I was in the hospital.

Ron and I had a great talk while I received my platelet transfusion. (Platelets, by the way, are not red, they look like *turkey gravy*. "Where's the mashed potatoes?" I asked the nurse. Humor, always good to have.) We talked about mind and visualization healing, something he tapped into to help with his own past health issues. He told me he'd teach me some techniques, and I look forward to that help. We were at the infusion center about two hours, and off back home, where Ron had planned to cook a meal.

And what a meal it was! The menu was salmon marinated in garlic and dill, accompanied by peach-butter compote. On the side were sautéed spinach, roasted rosemary potatoes, and Rachel's yummy stir-fried rice (except it wasn't rice, it was quinoa). Quite decadent and divine!

My energy level at this point was continuing to decline, and fatigue was settling in. But that afternoon—the cards from my family, spending time with Ron, and then this amazing meal—was a gift brought to me at the right time to buoy me through my physical state. And, of course, my greatest gift was seeing my husband's beautiful face walk through the door Friday night, just in time to enjoy the scrumptious meal Ron prepared for us, and just in time to scoop me up in his strong arms and soothe my weary soul.

This morning, I was scheduled to receive one unit of blood at Sky Ridge. I did not sleep well. Fever, gas pain, and fatigue continued to plague me. The fatigue is so great, it almost makes you restless. Another paradox. I was really frustrated and tired, and the idea of going through four to six more cycles of this crap made me angry and sad all at once. I was walking upstairs with my hand over my tear-streaked eyes, and in my silent frustration, I didn't see Chris sitting there. I let gravity take me and I just fell in his arms, sobbing. My husband, my strength, my savior. I can tell this just rips him apart to see his wife in physical and emotional pain. He held me tight and let me have my moment, there on his shoulder, on our stairs, in silence.

We finished getting ready and headed to Sky Ridge. The transfusion went well, but I catnapped through most of the three hours we were there; it was difficult keeping my eyes open. Back home, I felt like a zombie and curled up in bed for a couple of hours. Chris went to the grocery store and picked up some things to help my digestion: DanActive, Activia, and Maalox. The DanActive and Activia seemed to soothe my raw stomach. I called a friend who had wanted to stop by over the weekend and left her a message that I just wasn't up for visitors. I later called my sister, who was planning to come over to help with dinner, and told her the same, even though I could greatly use a sister hug. She understood.

It was just me and Chris today, and I needed some down time to rest and to spend with him. He had been out of town and missed his wife. He really hates being away and not completely in charge and overseeing Project Barb, but at the same time, he is beginning to enjoy this new job; it is offering him some new and exciting opportunities and challenges that so fit his talents. I have never been more proud or more in love with him than I am right now, if that were even possible. There is so much more of me to give him; I cannot wait until I am fully healthy and capable of giving all to him that he has so unconditionally given me. He is my life. What better gift is that?

And so I count each blessing, each gift. This challenge and struggle in my life goes on, and while I will go ahead and feel the crappiness that I feel, and have my little pity parties, they do not last long, and neither will this cancer. Balance. Equilibrium. Yin and Yang. Ebb and Flow. Cause and Effect. Laws of Nature. There is just so much to be said for the simple statement "things have a way of working themselves out."

One final gift was in that package I received from Cousin Kathy yesterday. Another handmade perfection, which I will frame. It said:

Love
Quietly covers all things,
Believes all things,
Hopes all things,
Endures all things.
—1 Corinthians 13:7

Mojo

When you're weary, feeling small. I love that Simon and Garfunkel song. "Bridge Over Troubled Water" was going through my head a lot yesterday, calming my soul. Sunday morning came, and Cat Stevens was the voice in my head singing "Morning Has Broken." Such great lyrics, so soothing. *Mine is the sunlight, mine is the morning.*

The ju-ju juice is working. Or mojo. Take your pick; it's perking me up. I awoke much better than the previous day, and Chris and I traveled again to Sky Ridge for the last unit of ju-ju, my mojo in a bag. This transfusion went well, and back home, I felt alive and close to normal again. I managed through eight loads of laundry—fully resting in between, of course—while I caught reruns of Food Network's *Next Food Star*, which culminated in a win—tonight a star is born. And later, our masseuse came by to give me and Chris massages. We had recently reconnected with her after she left working at our chiropractor's office. Chris and I decided that this therapy needed to be back in our lives, with him in a new job, me fighting cancer. Nothing's better than relaxing and transcending your body for sixty minutes to heal and rejuvenate.

I am nearly through all my cycle two drug treatment days—only one more day of taking prednisone. Yay! Then seven full days of rest. I am so very excited! I don't know how long the chemo drugs stay in the body breaking down the cells, but I am hopeful my body will restore itself during the seven "off" days and get ahead of producing its own white and red blood cells and platelets, ready to be in a stronger fighting position to start cycle three. Because cycle four is my goal. Done. No more cancer cells. It's ambitious, I know, and I probably won't be able to convince my doctor to go ahead and take that PET scan two cycles early to see that the cancer has been eradicated. But it is good to have goals, something to shoot for. I expect to have a good week ahead of me. I'll start walking again in the morning, look into yoga and some other healing remedies to aid my body during this time. I feel on top of the world.

Nightmares and Sunrises

"You freaked me out," I said as I awoke to find my brother standing over my bed, looking at me with concern. "I didn't know it was you."

"Are you okay?" he asked.

"Yes, why? Was I dreaming?" I was a little groggy.

"You were *screaming* in your sleep," he said. "It woke me up in the other room, so I came to check on you."

Perhaps I should have shut my bedroom door, and my screams may not have woken him in the night. I glanced at the clock; it was 1:30 am. I had gone to bed just after midnight.

"Oh, yeah, I do that sometimes. I didn't think I was having a nightmare, but I guess I was. I'm fine," I said.

"You were loud. I didn't know what was wrong." He paused, still with a look of worry. "Okay, as long as you're alright." He didn't seem convinced.

Even though I had told him he freaked me out when I opened my eyes to see him standing there looking at me, how freaky must it be to hear your sister, who is sick, screaming in the middle of the night? That thought didn't occur to me until later; all I was thinking at that moment was *Cool, I finally hit some good REM sleep.*

I am a screamer, a yeller in the bedroom (minds out of the gutter, please). It doesn't happen often, but on occasion, when dreaming or having a nightmare, I will scream in my sleep. The first time I was made aware of this was about ten years ago. I was on a girls' vacation in San Francisco with one of my friends, a night owl. One night, she stayed up watching TV in our hotel room, while I dozed off. The next thing I know, she's shaking me awake, apparently alarmed at my screaming outburst from deep in my sleep. I recall that I was dreaming that someone or something was chasing me and I was very scared. Oftentimes, these dreams are quite real. I feel I'm in a semiconscious state—a place of awareness and deep sleep—and there is some presence in my room that I can feel and sometimes see, but I can't quite make out who it is or why he or she is there. I try talking to the presence, asking him what he wants and telling him to go away. I know, this is all classic boogeyman stuff, but my brain thinks it's really happening. I try communicating to the "thing," and when it doesn't respond or go away, my flight/fight response kicks in and I begin yelling and screaming. My sister, who has had similar experiences, told me she saw a documentary on TV about this phenomenon actually being some kind of sleep disorder. This is how some stories about alien abduction come in to being (seriously). While I don't think there's any *Invasion of the Body Snatchers* going on in my bedroom, it is hard to admit that as an adult, I still have scary nightmares. Chris was concerned when he witnessed this "condition" firsthand early in our relationship but has since learned to simply wake me up and bring me back to consciousness so the boogeyman doesn't take me away. Imagine this condition with a chemo-hazed brain.

I awoke the next morning at the usual 6:00 am, and my stomach wanted food. It's used to the early morning routine. Feed me, Seymour. I got up, happy that I didn't have to take any prednisone. Chris had been the one attending to the outdoor flowers all summer, and I realized with him out of town the night before, I didn't water them. I went out to our backyard and greeted and watered each plant. The morning was cool and crisp, and I felt so alive. So good, in fact, that I decided to take a walk versus feed the tummy.

Michael was stirring upstairs, so I let him know of my adventure. "Where are you going? How long will you be?" he asked. I told him my route and to come look for me if I wasn't back in about thirty minutes.

I hadn't been walking in more than two weeks, so I was thrilled at my energy level that morning. I was like a kid on a bike for the first time, walking up my street, scooping the fresh morning air into my lungs, taking such delight in my feet moving in rhythm—one, two; one, two. Each breath of air was a breath of life and sunshine goodness into my soul. The street I live on rises at a slight incline for about five blocks, and before I knew it, I had hit the apex of the climb without any trouble breathing. I was suddenly overcome with emotion and just broke into tears realizing that *my body was working*. The endorphins kicked in, I quickened my pace, and my heart sang as I rounded the corner and headed toward the park. I was now walking toward the east and watching the sun rise. And what a sunrise it was. A large, gray cloud lay at the horizon, in the shape of a fluffy pancake or frittata. (I was getting hungry, and breakfast was on the brain.) Above and below the cloud, the sun's rays were spanning out, seemingly reaching toward me. And right in the middle of the gray pancake-shaped cloud was a break, enough for the sun to radiate through in brilliant pink and orange bursts of light. It was gorgeous—nature's beauty and wonder unfolding in front of me.

The day continued with more positive news from my blood results. All counts rebounded from the transfusions over the weekend. Yay! I was now free until next week, Tuesday, when cycle three begins. The joy!

It was short-lived, however. Chris came home from his trip just as my body was crashing early last night. I was so thrilled to see him but was starting to notice I couldn't carry on a conversation with him for very long; my breath was labored, and the tenderness I had felt in some of my lymph nodes earlier in the day was getting more pronounced, especially under my left armpit. My muscles were getting achy, and fatigue was settling in. I told Chris what I was feeling and he said, "Please call your doctor." I was disappointed. My day had started so amazingly well, the counts were great, and here I was staring at my cell phone not wanting to make yet another after-hours call to my doctor. I just sat there with my head in my hand, listless, pissed. My doctor was on call, and when we spoke, there was an air of concern in his voice over my swollen glands, and he asked me to come in the next day for him to examine me. He theorized that since I stopped taking prednisone the day before, perhaps my body was reacting to that. Prednisone, that happy steroid, is an anti-inflammatory, and maybe I was experiencing the pains of inflammation with the sudden stop of the dosage. "Take two Tylenol," he said, "and call my office in the morning and come on in so I can check you out."

I awoke this morning after a good night's sleep still very fatigued and with pain in my left armpit. As the day goes on, however, my energy level is rising, the aches subsiding. I have an appointment to see the doctor today at two o'clock. This roller coaster is not a fun ride. Thank goodness for yesterday's beautiful sunrise.

Reading the Teacups
August 2008

I was glad to see my doctor Wednesday afternoon, and since then, I have been feeling pretty well overall. He didn't have any concern about the tenderness in my lymph nodes in my neck, and he told me what to look for if I get an infection at any of my surgery sites: the lymph node biopsy area under my left armpit and where the port is in my chest. The inflammation I must have experienced is for the most part gone, but I continue to feel soreness at the biopsy site, which forty-eight hours later on Friday afternoon prompted me to call the doctor's office and speak with the nurse. *Shouldn't the soreness be gone?* They weren't concerned and told me to continue to watch for red streaks around the site, hotness to touch, a temperature over 100.5, and if I start to feel really bad. Basically, cool your jets, missy. I still struggle as to when to call or not. I mean, is it multiple choice—if you have two or more of the above then call—or does it only count if I hit all four?

Today, Saturday, the pain in that same area persists. It really hurts. I did feel "really bad" when I awoke this morning, but no temperature. The site was pink but not red and warm but not hot. The mystery is like trying to grill a steak: how would you like that cooked—rare, medium rare, or well done? The only thing I can figure is that eight weeks after the biopsy surgery, the nerve endings are beginning to heal or scar tissue is forming underneath the incision, and that is the pain I am feeling. Whatever it is, it hurts, and my doctor doesn't seem concerned. "Take two Tylenol" is the standard response. I can manage two Tylenol. After having breakfast and resting, the feeling "really bad" is gone, and I am doing well. Aargghh, the roller coaster!

Despite the roller-coaster ride and crashing a couple of times, this has been a very good week. My brother Michael was here Monday through Thursday afternoon, while Chris was either out of town or had to be at off-site meetings. My mom and Michael's daughter, my sweet niece Elsa, were here for part of the time as well. Michael then passed the "sitter" baton over to my very good friend Alex, who stayed with me Thursday evening and most of Friday. I had other social visitors as well. Wednesday night, my good friend Amy and her husband, Ludi, cooked a splendid dinner for me, Chris, and Michael, and brought some great laughter into our home. Thursday morning, Ron came over to walk me through a healing and meditative exercise in spiritual visualization— incredible! That night, a few of my book club girlfriends were over for dinner. Again, another great evening filled with laughter, sharing great stories, and just living life. I am lucky these family members and friends have the flexibility within their daily lives to be with me during this time. Chris is comforted knowing I'm in good hands while he establishes his new role. I am so pleased to see him exuberant and enthusiastic about his new venture. And Chris's mom arrived this afternoon for a two-week stay. We are so grateful to have her help, and I am looking forward to spending time getting all kinds of good motherly love from her.

Last evening, I was thinking of this incredible network of mine, and an image of a teacup and saucer flashed in my mind. That image made me immediately think of my cousin Kathy, whom Chris and I visited in Austin, Texas, this past April. We had never been to Austin, and at last year's reunion, Kathy had extended the invitation for us to come visit her and her husband, Tom, in the "little blue dot in the middle of a big red state," as she described it. I was intrigued.

During our visit, I noticed Kathy's collection of beautiful and ornate teacup sets on display in her curio cabinet. She explained that the collection started with one set many years ago, and she added to it by purchasing pieces as she visited places around the globe. Soon, she had family and friends seeking out sets to add to her collection. Now, I am not the collector type—although if you saw the junk drawer in my kitchen, you would beg to differ—but viewing Kathy's display of beautiful teacups and saucers and listening to her wonderful stories of how they came to be part of her collection, I was in awe of the spirit and life that was brought forth by these gorgeous objects. It was a whole level of beauty that I had not appreciated until that moment.

And so last night, I was counting my blessings for the day and week, which has become quite routine for me throughout this journey, when that picture of a teacup and saucer flashed across my mind. And as I examined that image more carefully, I realized that life is like one of those precious teacups in Kathy's curio cabinet—beautiful, full of wonderful stories, unique, and carefully crafted by its creator as if in a bold expression of its soul to be shared with all who would come in contact with it, and at the same time fragile, delicate, and necessitating careful handling to maintain that beauty and expression, its wholeness.

And I thought about myself as that teacup and the delicacy and fragility of my current state, while at the same time, I have the freedom to express my soul, my truest self, here in this journal and share it with family and friends. If I am the teacup, then the saucer represents my husband and family. It (they) holds me, the teacup, and lets me rest upon it (them). It is my support. We are a match; we go together, and we stay together. And if the saucer represents family, then it is my friendships that are the tea—they fill my cup with warmth, energy, and calmness; they are the soothing liquid to my heart and soul. Teas come in all sorts of colors and flavors, and like friendships, you either enjoy a wide variety if your tastes are many or drink that one favorite flavor you love, but you sample many to see which ones you enjoy and end up sticking with the ones that you know and trust.

I don't know if Kathy's collection is meant for filling with tea, but the utility the cups represent is still there. And now it is easy for me to see that connection, and I understand why that image of a teacup and saucer popped into my brain at that moment while I counted my blessings. Forrest Gump's mother may have given him sage advice with the "life is like a box of chocolates" tagline and the you-never-know-what-you-get uncertainty to it all, but for me, thinking of Kathy's beautiful collection has made life's mystery a little clearer. And the next time I have a cup of tea, I will enjoy it with complete contentment and in full appreciation and honor of my life, my family, and my friends.

A Bump in the Path

"Eewww, grossssss!" That is what I said out loud as pus started pouring from the incision under my left armpit.

What is it about me that doctors don't take me seriously? When I say I'm sick, please find out what is wrong; don't tell me I'm depressed. When I say I am in pain, please don't pat me on the head like I'm a little girl and tell me not to worry about it. *People, listen to me!* I must either look like or behave like a hypochondriac or somehow not communicate strongly enough that something is wrong.

Last week, I was in my oncologist's office showing him the painful incision site. *It hurt!* Doesn't look like it's infected, he says. On Friday, I call in, saying I am still in pain there. Is that right, two months after my surgery? "Well," the nurse says, "sometimes it takes weeks for the biopsy site to heal, and you can still feel soreness." Even though she consulted my doctor, they didn't think it was serious enough to see me for a second time on the same issue that week. By Sunday night, I am calling my doctor about the topic again, asking if I can take Vicodin, the pain is so great. No, I report, I don't have that magic frickin' 100.5 temperature, and no, I don't have happy red streaks streaming down from the site or down the back of my arm. "Sure," he says, "go ahead and take Vicodin every four hours." Just fine. (Vicky helped greatly—made me very loopy, which I am sure was quite impressive in front of my mother-in-law. I even made loopy phone calls.)

I woke up yesterday morning to find that one end of my incision site has now developed into a nice, big whitehead that looks as though it's going to burst like Old Faithful any moment. I called the nurse's voice mail line at my doctor's office. Why bother trying to talk to anyone directly? Who would take me seriously, anyway? You could hear the smirk in my message:

> I am calling again about the painful incision under my left armpit, which has been swollen and painful now for six days. No, I don't have any other symptoms, but just wanted you to know I have a giant pimple on it and it looks like it wants to break free any moment. That tells me it's infected. I am scheduled to be there tomorrow to start cycle three, but thought I should let

you know about this little development in case you wanted to call me back and maybe see me today.

I got a call back in an hour. "Barb, how soon can you come in today?"

At the office, the nurse took a look at the area. "Yeah, that looks bad." (Ya think?) Then my doctor: "Yeah, that's an abscess in a couple of your stitches. I'll prescribe you some antibiotics to take three times a day over the next ten days to clear this up."

"What about tomorrow?" I ask. "I'm supposed to start cycle three. Do I still come in?"

"Yes. I'll want to check the area first," says the doc.

The nurse told me to put warm, moist heat on the site to draw out some of the infection. I left the office happy to have any answer, but geez, could we maybe have started the antibiotics sooner than yesterday?

And now back to ew, gross! I am applying the warm, moist heat with a washcloth to the infected area early yesterday evening, and out gushes the creamy pus. It oozes from the edge of the incision down the left side of my torso in a streak like a rabid dog's drool—same consistency, but the color is light puke-green. I wipe away streak number one, and another oozing, infected glop of drool spits out. Wipe. Then another. Wipe. Then another. This goes on for an hour.

Meanwhile, our good friends Derek and Liz are downstairs, having stopped by to cook us dinner. I don't know what to do with this draining crap. Then Chris checks in on me with beer in hand. He is a masher of bumps. He sees a zit, and it has no chance with him. I am not a masher; I prefer to let these things work their way out of the body on their own time. He is quite tempted to help me flush and mash out all the greenish gunk until it bleeds. "No, thank you, honey. Besides, I am platelet-challenged, remember?" I don't want to bleed all over the place.

I finally made a call to the doctor's office. The doc on call was the head honcho, the practice owner. You mention this guy's name to anyone in the medical field, and he is like a god. God, by the way, needs to be paged twice. I've talked to him a couple of times in the office; he knows his stuff. When he finally calls me after page number two, I explain to him what has transpired the last few days, and he says, "What? Your incision from two months ago is abscessing? That's not right." (Exaaaaactly. That is what I have been trying to tell people, that my incision should not be causing me any problems eight weeks later!) Anyway, how the heck do I dress or clean this vile, draining cesspool—with peroxide? He tells me to stop putting moist heat on it, do not clean with anything but mild soap and water, let it drain naturally, do not force out the infected liquid. Dress it loosely with gauze and tape to allow more drainage—it is good that it is draining, he says. "What about cycle three tomorrow?" I ask. "I kinda need my white blood cells to heal this infection, don't I?" He says, "Your doctor will look at it tomorrow. If your counts are whacked out, we might give you an antibiotic intravenously."

I call Chris into our bathroom. "Honey, I need gauze. Can you go out and buy some for me?" He leaves me in the bathroom. I am half naked, pus oozing, and after a few minutes, I hear him laughing from somewhere in the house. Why was he still here—did he send his mom to get the gauze? I call his cell phone. "Honey, is your mom getting the gauze?" He says no, he hasn't left yet. I lose it. *"Get me the gauze now!"* When you have cancer, your fuse is very short. And I have been sitting on the edge of my bathtub, dripping, for more than an hour, while my husband is sipping a beer and laughing. I do not find humor in the situation. And anxiety and fear are creeping into my thoughts—people die from complications such as this. Chris's hairstylist had told him recently that her father had Hodgkin's lymphoma and died years ago. Granted, he was in his seventies, but he died not from the cancer, but from an infection that entered through his port. His body was so immune deficient from the chemo treatments that it couldn't recover. This is no trifling matter. I'm truly panicking at that moment.

Liz comes into my room. She hasn't seen me this frustrated and irritable before. A mother of two young boys, she knows how to calm and soothe, and before you know it, she has me cooing like a baby at her magic touch. Did she *Love and Logic* me? Maybe. Chris finally arrives with the gauze, and together, the two of them patch me up well enough that I can go downstairs to join Liz's husband Derek and Chris's mom and we can finally have dinner together.

Oh, and dinner! So spectacular! Derek, an amazing cook, served up grilled halibut atop saffron rice, topped with crabmeat and a drizzled corn cream-sauce reduction. This family-and-friend network of mine rolls out the red carpet treatment. We ate and enjoyed each other's company and stories. My broken record will repeat throughout this journal and the rest of my life how lucky, lucky, blessed, blessed I am for these beautiful souls in my and Chris's lives. My panicking moment in the bathroom is light years away.

It is now day one of cycle three. Chris sweetly held his sick wife a little longer this morning before he prepared for his business trip. His mom and one of my best friends, Jackie (who is currently visiting me from out of town), accompanied me to my doctor's appointment. My blood was drawn and I awaited the counts. They were good! I felt great, and had I not had the darn painful incision area the past few days, I would have felt like a million dollars. My doctor inspected the infected site. Most of the pain is now gone, I told him, and I have drained a lot out of it, but it is still hard in some places, and the oozing continues. He made the decision to give me a week off from chemo to give the infection time to clear up. He said the chemo drugs I would have received this week would only knock down my white blood count, which is what I need to help fight the infection. I suspected that would be the case.

I am grateful for the extra time off, as I do not want my body to crash again from the chemo while it is trying to heal a huge infection. I'm also a little worried that delaying treatment might slow any progress against the disease, but I feel in my heart that much of my body is already healed from the cancer cells. My white blood cell count is in a normal, healthy range, while my red blood cell counts are below normal, but still in "Barb-normal" range. My platelets are finally in normal range, four times what the Barb-normal range has been. My body is producing its own cells, which tells me the cancer cells in my bone marrow are diminishing. Additionally, my digestive system has been stabilized and fairly normal the past few days, indicating that new cells in this area are also reproducing. Cycle four, you are within reach!

A Little Reprieve

The future belongs to those who believe
in the beauty of their dreams.
—Eleanor Roosevelt

That quote was handwritten by our waitress on our breakfast check this morning. How perfectly timed that message was, capping an already perfect morning, and foreshadowing a perfect day for me—the best I've had since being diagnosed, and quite possibly the best I have felt physically this entire year. I had a good night's sleep for once—seven hours—although I did wake with a dull headache, something that I noticed has been happening with some frequency, particularly during my off-chemo days.

Jackie and I walked early this morning, and later we went out to breakfast with my mother-in-law. I decided I wanted to drive, which was a surprising announcement to my houseguests—I had not driven since before the emergency room visit two months ago. I'm sure they were nervous. I got behind the wheel of the car and couldn't believe how freeing it felt as I pulled out of the garage onto the street. It was like being back on skis after taking a season off. I was keenly aware of the vehicle, the road, and how my body was controlling and responding to the hundreds of stimuli coming at me as I navigated the car onward. I couldn't believe how much I had missed driving! We arrived at the restaurant, and as I looked for a place to park on the street, there was only one slot and I had to parallel park. I attacked that challenge with such finesse, I felt on top of the world! And the restaurant, Gaia Bistro, recommended by a good friend, was awesome. Quite possibly this could be my most favorite breakfast place. And then the nicely handwritten note from our waitress—how perfect.

After breakfast, we went shopping. I was looking for more lounge-type clothing to wear for my expanding waistline. We spent a couple of hours shopping, and I purchased some great comfy pieces. I couldn't believe the energy I had; I was out nearly six hours today and didn't crash and burn. We all had a terrific day, us girls.

This extra time off is giving me some buffer days, and I feel I am definitely on the road to recovery. The doctors will still want me to complete as many cycles as possible to ensure the cancer is gone, but the treatment is working, my body is responding, and I can tell that it wants so much to heal and repair itself. So does its occupier.

Earlier this morning, as I changed the dressing on my infected biopsy area, I noticed on the dressing two tiny, fine hairs. Aha! Those two little unsuspecting hairs are what caused the infection—ingrown hairs. They didn't have anywhere to go underneath the sewn-up incision, and probably didn't start growing until after the surgery. Who knows when they started to fester with infection, but that is what caused so much misery and goo the past few days. This morning, there was very little, if any, swelling, and the site was just a little tender, but clearly on its way to being healed. Now, other than this darned headache, I feel terrific.

I am extremely hopeful about my full recovery, and very determined. I believe in the beauty of my dreams. The future is mine.

From the Inside Out

I'm a little sad tonight, trying to find some inspiration to write, and having difficulty putting my heart into it. I miss my husband. A crack in this blissful marital veneer is starting to show some imperfections beneath the surface, as we both struggle with the situation of my cancer and his new job. The pressure of these two life events is creating tension, which is spilling out into our conversations and stressing us both. He wants to be here with me, but his main focus has to be success in his new job. I am focusing on getting 100 percent healthy but miss having him by my side. We have gone from spending so much time together when we both worked in the same office, to now figuring out how to master our lives separately. Each of these life events requires the entirety of our undivided attention, and we are both going it alone at a time when we need each other most.

We did not have a good conversation tonight; he said I made him feel guilty. It was not at all my intention, and I suspect he feels a good dose of that already without my help. Even though our journeys seem separate, at the end of the day, we each understand that what we do individually is for the other, so that we are free to enjoy our lives together unencumbered by my ill health and with some financial freedom to enjoy life. That is what we are working toward, and there is no one more important to him than me, and vice versa. I made him feel bad, and I am sad for that. I love this man with all my heart and soul. I need to learn how to appreciate him more. There is so much I need to learn on this journey of mine.

After my most splendid day yesterday, last night brought another interesting discovery. Before I went to bed, I changed out the dressing on my infected biopsy site. I put a warm, moist washcloth on it for a few minutes, as I saw there was some gunk that needed to come forth. After wiping out some of the whitish, cottage-cheese-like goo, I could see something that looked almost black trying to work its way out. By the end of my cleaning session, five of these pieces of black stitches (as I thought they were), came out of the incision site, leaving a half-inch hole. I was alarmed at this discovery; I thought the stitches were supposed to dissolve. I also recalled seeing the same sort of piece on the floor of my shower that morning. I'd wondered at the time if it came from my body somehow. I didn't know what it was and thought it odd that it was on my shower floor. I saved these pieces, six in all.

Concerned about this development and worried about the hole in my incision, I knew I needed to call the doctor in the morning. But I decided not to call my oncologist. His specialty is blood and cancer, not surgery. Yes, better to seek out the surgeon who performed the biopsy and stitched me up. I called the surgeon's office the next morning and was told he was out, but that the physician assistant, Tracy, wanted to see me to check things out. I remember meeting her in the hospital before I had the surgery, and she also visited me the next day after the procedure to follow up. She was very nice.

In the exam room, Tracy asked for details of what was going on with the site, and as I relayed the events to her, she took notes on her laptop. At one point, she stopped me and said that I was a very good storyteller. Finally, a health care provider who is listening to me! She said it's very unusual for surgical sites to abscess. She confirmed that the stitches should have dissolved by now. I told her I brought them in to show her, and at first, she didn't seem interested in seeing them, saying, "That's okay; I know what they look like. But since you have them, let me take a peek." When I showed them to her, Tracy's eyes widened and she said, "Oh, those are your clips! I have never seen them rejected by a body before!" She was genuinely surprised. I didn't know what she meant by *clips*. She explained that clips are made of titanium, a metal that the body does not typically reject, and they are used very routinely in surgeries. These were used to clamp off the blood vessels that surrounded the lymph node removed for biopsy. Surgical clips allow the blood vessels to heal, then scar tissue forms over them and they stay in the body. She read in the notes from my surgery that multiple clips were used in the procedure. Stunned by this information, I asked her if there were any others in there and would my body continue to reject these? Unlikely, she said, and even if there were, it was not something they would open me up to fish around for. If there were more, she surmised that my body would eventually force those out as well. Tracy was a little excited by this discovery, a first in her nine-year experience, and she said she couldn't wait to share it with the surgeon. *Great, I'm a guinea pig,* I thought.

Tracy examined the incision and poked around the open hole left by the expelled clips. She said it was healing just fine. When I asked her if two small hairs I found in the pus may have caused the infection, she replied no and that it was definitely the clips. Most unusual, because they were under layers of skin and muscle at the lymph node site and my body wrestled and maneuvered these objects out on its own, *Like a geyser,* I thought. Tracy's bedside manner was so refreshing, and the information she shared was of such tremendous help that I left there quite relieved, confident that the area was going to heal completely.

Taking Ownership

It is the eve of cycle three. I haven't written in a few days, the longest drought in my journal thus far. Very odd that I would get writer's block now, considering how fantastic I have been feeling the past several days despite a healing infection and throbbing headaches. Tracy, the surgeon's physician assistant, called me yesterday to follow up, and I reported that I'm doing well and the site is also looking good. She told me that the surgeon was just as shocked as she was when she told him my body rejected the titanium clips, and he wants to make sure I get in touch with them should the biopsy site give me any further problems. I told her I would, but that comment made me a little suspicious—was the surgeon concerned that there were more little titanium gems awaiting their time for escape? Hmmm.

The headaches I have been having may be due to my grinding my teeth at night. Several days ago, my sister (who should have become a doctor) told me if I'm waking up with a headache, then I am probably having issues with TMJ (temporomandibular joint and muscle). She has worked in the dental field her entire career and knows a thing or two about TMJ. She gave me some isometric exercises to do morning and night with my jaw. The exercises have actually helped alleviate my headaches; that, plus wearing my night guard the past three nights—a night guard I have had for more than three years but have rarely used.

So, on the eve of cycle three, I feel great, have had several days of good, consistent energy, and have walked almost daily. I expect to go into tomorrow's chemo treatment with decent blood counts, and I also anticipate an easier cycle than the last one. I will be surprised and sorely disappointed if my counts are not good.

Nine weeks after my hospital stay and the ultimate diagnosis, there are some notable observations about how my having cancer has impacted those around me. Overall, the outpouring of support and love from everyone has been tremendous and leaves me speechless. At the same time, though, I am also struck by how a few of my closest friends seemingly don't know how to approach me or have been AWOL in my journey, not reading or keeping up on my writings, or worse yet, not sending one get-well wish, whether by phone, e-mail, card, or otherwise.

Cancer is this big, mysterious black hole for many people, even though just about every one of us has been affected by this disease in some fashion, having friends, coworkers, or family members who have survived or lost their lives to it. The very word is scary or sad, and maybe for some, having cancer may seem so incomprehensible that they themselves may be unsure how to manage through a challenge such as mine. This fear of having to face, recognize, or ask themselves the tough questions can sometimes create an invisible wedge that almost paralyzes a relationship. Then there are times when my challenge reminds others of a very tragic event. Such is the case with my mother-in-law. She told me of the painful struggle her own mother went through with bladder cancer twenty-two years ago, which ultimately took her life. My experience seems to conjure up those painful memories as if they happened yesterday.

I think about how I would react if the shoe were on the other foot. Would I be the one extending myself as so many have, or would I stand on the sidelines, paralyzed, unsure how to react? Would I be generous in my love and support, or would I disappear? For me, being the cancer patient and living the experience almost ensures that I will not be on the sidelines should cancer or any other challenge strike down someone close to me. But I do recall when the human resources manager at my work, Vicki, lost her battle to breast cancer this past spring, after a two-year fight. I remember her struggle with the disease, her contagious optimism as she battled through several months of chemo, and the joy we felt when she went into remission. Then the cancer came raging back, and within months, it took her life. *I think about her every day.* She was a tremendous spirit in our office, a great listener and mentor to those who sought her advice, as I did many times; there was never a bad time or wrong question with Vicki. I was so deeply saddened by her struggle, but I was pretty much on the sidelines, somewhat paralyzed and unsure how I could help. I was told that in her final days, she was surrounded by the warmth and love of her family and she left this earth peacefully.

I don't know why cancer strikes, but I do know that it is not an automatic death sentence. I think for many of those on the outside who are uninformed about the disease, cancer equals death. *It doesn't.* For so many like me, it is a blessing in that it changes you forever, and almost always for the better. It forces you to look deep into your soul and challenges you to look at life differently. But I would never wish it on anyone; that is the paradox. If only we could look deep into our souls and view life differently or recognize it as more magnificent than our current struggles and stresses without facing cancer or any other event that would challenge us to the core—that is the miracle I would wish for everyone.

My mother-in-law asked me if I dreaded tomorrow. I told her no; in fact, I look forward to it. She looked a little perplexed by my answer. I welcome the treatment; it is getting me better, despite how lousy it makes me feel. There is no alternative. Refusing treatment would surely mean death, and dreading it (for me) means I don't have the right mental attitude to get through it. And getting through it is the goal, because on the other side is the rest of my happy, healthy life. That is where I want to be; that is where I will be. Don't take this pain from me and wear it so I don't have to feel it. I would not want anyone to feel this pain or go through this challenge, especially not for me. It is in me, and mine to bear, and I own it and will be rid of it so no one, including me, is burdened by it ever again.

CYCLE THREE

The Universe Is Calling

Spiritual Sensations

Two days into cycle three, and so far, no issues! I was a little tired after yesterday's session but bounced back later in the evening and awoke feeling great this morning. I had another slight allergic reaction to today's treatment, and we discovered the nurse did not slow down the IV drip of the chemo drug Etopiside (also called VP-16). They discovered during my earlier treatments that this particular drug causes my breakouts and the best way to minimize the allergic reaction is to slow down the rate at which the drug is being infused into my body (plus an infusion of Benadryl). That's been the reason for my longer chemo appointments, particularly on days one through three.

There is so much going on in the doctor's office, multiple patients going in and out, that you really need to keep on top of your own specific protocol, because as far as I can tell, each patient has a different cancer and treatment plan. When you enter the office, the first thing they do is check your vitals: weight, blood pressure, heart rate, and oxygen rate. I have lost about four pounds during my off time, probably due to losing excess water weight, getting some extra exercise, and really watching what I am eating—less comfort food, more organic protein and veggies, and cutting down on my sugar intake. The first several weeks, I just wanted to gorge, but now I am learning that while it felt great to eat whatever I wanted, I paid the price in gas pain and discomfort, plus an additional ten pounds. The doctor and nurses prefer you gain weight versus losing it, but I am listening to my body and wanting to do what's best. Thankfully, neither the disease nor the treatment is controlling this aspect of my life—I am. My blood pressure during previous office visits had been borderline high and now seems back to normal the last two days. My heart rate is still a little high, around ninety beats per minute, but it's not in the hundreds as it was during cycle two. I'd like to see that go down by ten to fifteen beats, but it's not alarming to the staff. My oxygen rate has always been strong, between 94 and 98 percent lung capacity.

After the vitals check, you are taken back to the sitting area—some are private, other areas are shared by two patients—where you recline in a chair and settle in for your treatment. Patients are allowed one guest, and you can watch TV or DVDs, listen to music (through headphones), or sit and visit with your guest. There is some interaction between patients, mostly between those who have been coming in for treatments for a long time. (An older lady I sat next to one time was in for her thirty-second cycle; my treatment plan is only supposed to be six to eight cycles.) Most of the patients are in their sixties or seventies. I have noticed a few new faces the past couple of days; most of these faces are younger.

My blood was drawn yesterday and today. The counts drawn on day one were solid numbers and much better than the level I started at in cycle two. Today's counts were mixed: white blood cells jumped up, while red blood cells came down about 10 percent—still in decent shape, but I will definitely need to keep an eye on it. After day two, my energy is stronger than it was yesterday, when I had to take a two-hour nap. No nap necessary today! I am so far encouraged by my body's response to this third round—no signs yet of infected hangnails or mouth ulcers; the stomach is a little bloated, but no gas pains. I am hopeful the roller-coaster ride will not be so wild this time.

Chris's mom has been here since the beginning of August and has been a great help and loving support. She told me tonight she is glad to be here to see firsthand that I am handling things so well. She has a peace of mind she didn't have before. I can imagine it is difficult to picture what I am going through via phone calls and my Web site. Two weeks is a long time to be away from your home and routine, particularly with issues going on back home: Chris's dad is recovering from a workplace injury to his foot, and Chris's grandfather is in rehabilitation after having hip replacement surgery the other day. Chris's aunt is also facing surgery tomorrow, not to mention that his mom is taking time away from work to be with us. There is a lot of sacrifice going on for us.

Our only issue has been food. During this visit, my change from eating comfort food to healthy food has thrown her off a bit, but we are managing through it. My mother-in-law is from the South, where eating comfort food is a ritual. Finding and preparing healthy food is unfamiliar territory. But she is an amazing baker. Last week, she made two delicious cakes, one of them a favorite of ours—red velvet cake. This week I backed off on the sweets. It was difficult but something I felt my body was ready to do. Cancer loves sugar, so they say.

Chris is on his way home tonight. Next week he travels again, this time all week. It would have been my off week between treatments, but because my cycle three was delayed due to the infection, he will be traveling while I am still receiving treatments. Because of that, I had to arrange coverage while Chris is gone. He really does not like for me to be alone when he travels. My family and friends to the rescue once again, bless them all. I do believe I am on the upswing, and that by the off week of cycle three, I will be—expect to be—fairly independent of this help (if I can only convince my husband!).

I am comforted each and every day by the love, prayers, and support from family, friends, and even strangers! From my family network across the country, there are multiple church congregations mentioning me in their weekly prayers, so people I've never met are acknowledging my plight and sending me positive vibes. And believe me, I feel all of this, I really do. The prayers, e-mails, phone calls, and posts on my Web site give me such an amazing spiritual sensation—I wish I could bottle it and share it with the world.

One of the most amazing aspects of this journey is feeling like I have my own spiritual guru in Rick's partner, Ron. He has spent just two sessions with me thus far in meditation and visualization exercises, and they have been most helpful. Ron has an eclectic past, one which was once steeped in the spiritual, healing realm. Through my journey, he is tapping into that energy once again, and I am the lucky recipient.

Our first session began with Ron talking me into a relaxed state of mind. Next he asked me to visualize Mother Earth as this warm, honey-colored light entering through my toes and traveling up through my body toward my head, filling each crevice of my body with healing powers. He then had me imagine a bright white healing power from above entering the top of my head, mixing with the Mother Earth warm honey light and traveling down from my head, throughout my body, down to my toes. Next, he directed me to focus on my blood and had me visualize producing more blood cells, all of them happy, healthy cells racing through my body in exuberant bursts of energy, mixing with the

Mother Earth warm honey glow and the bright white healing power from above. He then had me turn my attention to my darker cells—the cancer cells in my body. He told me to see Mother Earth scooping up these cells and taking them out of my body back into the earth, where she will nourish them and take care of them. This amazing first session lasted about forty-five minutes. The best part is that he left me with the ability to access this visualization at any time.

During session two last week, after once again gently coaxing me into a relaxed state, Ron asked me to envision myself walking down stairs toward a misty haze with a bright light, which as I approached, turned out to be a gigantic library. He said this was a library of books of lives, if you will, and directed me to my book of life. As I flipped the pages of my book, he walked me through chapters of my life from my childhood to adulthood. The pages were filled with stories about my relationship with my siblings, my mom, and then, before Ron could even say it, I saw the chapter on my dad. Tears filled my eyes. My precious father, who passed eight years ago, how I miss him! We paused here as Ron let me reminisce and linger in the fond memories of my father. From there, he instructed me to turn to the chapter on my health—and the cancer. He had me visualize first embracing the cancer (figuratively) and then tearing out the pages. The next chapter, he said, was blank. He asked me to write it and asked me what I would name it. I said, "My new life." From there, he said, the possibilities were endless.

Ron brought me back out of the state of relaxation, and we had a wonderful discussion about what I experienced throughout the exercise. I explained to him that when he directed me to walk down the stairs, I didn't know if I was inside or outside, so the image in my mind kept changing from a dark wooden staircase with a rich, red carpet down the middle of the stairs, to a beautiful outdoor garden with steps made of stone. The walls were fluid, like liquid to match whichever stair I stepped down, sometimes paneled in beautiful, dark mahogany to match the wooden staircase, sometimes flanked by waterfalls flowing from majestic mountains into endless fields of wildflowers, complementing the stairs of stone. Even the library itself seemed fluid, and the shelves where he told me to find my book of life were swaying gently. I did not visualize myself as being in my body, but rather as a light of energy. And right before Ron mentioned my father, when I presciently knew that's where he was going, I saw my father, again, not in body, but as a warm glow wrapping around my energy, and on occasion from that warm glow, the shape of his smiling face would come forward to kiss my light energy. It was powerful and awesome and spiritual all at the same time.

All of these things—friends, family, strangers at churches, various stories being brought to me of people surviving and even the sad stories of those who lost their battle with cancer, the meditation, the books I am reading, this experience, *this journey*—inspire me, push me forward, and leave me more hopeful, peaceful, joyful, and full of so much love, *so alive*, that there is no room for doubt in my ability to recover. There is so much life I have yet to live; there is so much love I have yet to give.

A Broken Faith Restored

The weekend has been good so far. I am very tired. My hemoglobin count on Friday was low at 8.65 (a normal count is between 12 and 16), and I have to go in Monday for another lab check of my blood. It is possible I will need some mojo transfused on Tuesday. Such is the roller coaster. However, I am managing to stave off the other symptoms I felt during the first two cycles. Fatigue is really the only issue. I am not gorging out on food but instead am enjoying two to three solid meals a day with a couple of snacks, all pretty healthy. The stomach pains are all but gone, and no constipation. A combination of taking DanActive, Activia, and adding probiotics and Juice Plus to my diet seems to have had a positive impact on my stomach lining and digestion. I have a couple more days of the oral chemo, and of course, several days left of prednisone. We shall see what Monday's counts look like, but I do anticipate more red blood cell reduction; that is just what the chemo does.

My family was over here last night, which has become routine now each Saturday. I so enjoy having them all here, pitching in and preparing dinner for me, and just simply visiting and being together. Last night, Ron prepared a fabulous corn-lime chili and homemade chicken enchiladas—all to die for. And Mom brought over homemade blueberry and peach pies. Yum.

My dear friend Ilene, visiting from Phoenix, joined us for dinner. We have been friends for more than a dozen years but lost touch the past few years, as can sometimes happen when life events pull your focus elsewhere. I am very happy we have reconnected. We both lost our fathers several years ago, deaths that occurred within six months of each other, and I remember the time Ilene and I shared afterward, trying to piece together the emotional void our dads left.

Journaling is not new to me, but I stopped writing a few months after my father died. It was the year 2000, on June 30—he died exactly halfway through the first year of the new millennium. I last wrote in my journal on December 30 of that same year. At that time, I had been journaling off and on for several years. What started the writing was this path or spiritual journey I was on trying to discover myself, truth, God, answers, the universe (everything, basically). I did not journal daily; I usually picked up the pen whenever some life event had me perplexed. I wrote about topics that were searching in nature, like life beyond my own, past relationships and regrets, family and love. And as difficult as my life may seem now facing cancer, nothing has challenged me more than losing my father.

My father was the kindest, gentlest soul on the planet, so caring and full of love for me and my family. At the same time, he was a sad man who did not seem content with how his own life turned out, and was depressed toward the end. He was a smoker until heart issues started showing up at age forty-nine, and after three heart attacks, he finally gave up the nasty habit. He lived just fourteen more years, and ironically, his heart held up fine in his final hours. His lungs gave out, not because of any disease caused by smoking, such as emphysema (although I'm sure the years of smoking complicated the issue), but to an untreatable, untraceable lung disease: the same lung disease that claimed his uncle's life years prior to Dad's death, and also his eldest brother's life years later.

Interstitial lung disease was the diagnosis given to him in late April of 2000; it was terminal, and we were told he had two to five years to live. I will never forget when I got this news. My brother Rick called me at work to tell me. I remember the world stopping at that moment. Gawd, if only we had those two to five more years—but with complications from surgery and maybe his own resignation to stop fighting, he died two months later.

It was on Father's Day 2000 that I last saw Dad awake and conscious—and scared. He was back in the hospital, his lungs filling with fluid. The oxygen flowing through the mask on his face was cranked up to its highest level. All you could see were his bright blue eyes, wide and confused. "What is happening to me?" they were beseeching us. And it was on that day that I thought I saw him dying, his face blue and body limp, as I watched in horror as the medical team tried for what seemed like an eternity to get the breathing tube down his throat. He didn't die on Father's Day, thank goodness, but he never awoke and we never again saw those bright blue eyes. We had to make the painful decision to take him off life support two weeks later, his lungs shot, but his heart still going strong in the end. I wrote about this time that shook me to my core, losing my father, my rock, my support. And I lost the way on my journey; my faith was broken and so was my heart. After six months, I stopped writing altogether.

As sad and gut-wrenching as that time was, I did eventually regain my faith and hope in the world and the universe (although I did not pick up the pen again until now). Time is a gentle healer. And I also know that every happy, gleeful, successful, awe-inspired moment in my life since then has my father's hand on it. I feel his presence, I hear his voice, and I know he is with me right now, caressing my head, embracing my weariness, and kissing my light energy.

Hope

It is interesting how the mind plays tricks on you. I was convinced yesterday that my blood count would be lower than Friday's readings and I would then be in need of a transfusion today. The counts had been slowly dropping every day last week; by the weekend, I figured for sure the chemo would continue the effect of breaking down my cells. I was more tired, took more naps. It was a relief to see my red blood cell count actually held steady, although the white blood cells continue to drop. I received a shot of Procrit (Prudy, the gerbil ovaries) on Friday, but it takes up to one week for that shot to generate new red blood cell production. I am happy my body seems to be holding up well during this cycle; fatigue continues to plague me, but there is just no getting around having your cells torn down. The good news actually pepped me up, and I had more energy last night.

The prednisone is really affecting me this cycle in terms of physical appearance. I tipped the scale yesterday in the doctor's office. Twelve extra pounds in one week. My face, shoulders, midsection, and legs are all swollen. I am up in weight twenty pounds since beginning chemo and have gained back almost all the weight since I started losing it back in

November; however, I do expect this weight to continue to roller coaster. When I am off the prednisone and can start walking regularly again (red blood cell count needs to higher), the weight and water retention should subside some (dear God, I hope).

Chris and I had a great visit last night with our coworker and friend Deb, who brought by an exquisite meal of smoked salmon linguine. Phenomenal! Chris went out of town this morning and is back Thursday night. Today's sitter duties rested in the good hands of Ron. We had another amazing meditation session this afternoon. This journal and Ron are saving me thousands of dollars in psychotherapy! Brother Rick will be here for the overnight stay tonight, Chris still very insistent I am not alone during my chemo treatment days. And tomorrow, my sister will be here to take me to my day eight chemo appointment and hang with me for the day. At some point, and hopefully soon, I will be able to convince my adoring husband that I can manage fine without sitters and overnight stays. I do feel it is important to my recovery that I soon exercise independence, and my body is turning this corner to take that charge. I so appreciate his support and love and the absolute unwavering focus he puts on my well-being. Our time apart is not easy, but we feel this greater sense of the two us—our creative selves are being tapped to their fullest, and I feel there is nothing we won't be able to accomplish together.

I ebb and flow throughout my recovery from being so centrally focused on my body to reacting to and interacting with my surroundings and the energy flowing around me. As the observer and participant, I am trying to funnel my attention through the quagmire of this journey to heal and find purpose to my life. I say I want my life back, but not as it was before. I thought it was fulfilled, but it wasn't—I got sick. It was out of balance. I get energized and tired all at the same time trying to find answers, inspiration; the mental and physical exhaustion of it all wears me down. But I have to persevere, because if I don't, what is the purpose? Why am I here going through this, and what higher calling is out there for me? How do I use this life to a greater satisfaction and benefit for me, my husband, my family, friends, for others? So many things concern and interest me, so many questions swirling in my head trying to find definition in my fuzzy brain. How does someone go through cancer or any health challenge without good insurance, good family, friend, and support networks? How do they manage? I don't know where I would be without these blessings in my life. How can I help those less fortunate than myself; what form will that take? And what of this human race—the beauty and destruction of our diversities? How do we manage to live and inhabit this planet without more socially conscious awareness of each other and our resources? What has happened to the human face in corporate America? We forget our most important resource of human capital and focus more on shareholder wealth. Who are we trying to benefit? Who builds the wealth, who holds the wealth, who spends the wealth—would that be the very diverse human race that needs to be mindful of this planet?

Obviously my questions go from very personal, relating to my own experience, to global, and everything in between. I am not worried or fearful; to the contrary, I am most hopeful. I am swimming with possibilities to where I can begin this next new life of mine, healthy and contributing in ways that are so meaningful. I have a voice; I can organize and lead; I can write. It doesn't mean I abandon my old life; it means looking at how I can approach it differently and with more purpose. It means retooling and redirecting energy in a way that is more balanced and centered. It is facing the sun, arms outstretched, surrendered in the moment and finding peace, love and joy, and having faith in all things possible.

Humility

The body typically holds twenty units of blood, and so far, I have had eleven units infused. I have had more than half my blood replaced since June 9. That's so weird to think about. A body's *own* production of red blood cells lasts 120 days, while *infused* or *transfused* blood lasts only about thirty days. With the constant checking of my blood levels, I am starting to see patterns in how my body is reacting to the chemo, and together with my overall level of energy, these are the only indicators I have for how well I am healing. I would like to give myself a gold star. I haven't asked my doctor to grade me yet, but I can see he is pleased with my progress.

When receiving my day eight chemo treatment this past Wednesday, my sister, who was with me, commented that it seems my doctor is taking my feedback more seriously as he sees that I am listening to my body and am better able to participate in the decisions for my recovery, such as my giving the direction to go ahead and get blood yesterday. He was contemplating having me wait one more day to see how my counts looked before proceeding with an infusion, but I said, "Why bother when we both know I need the boost? Let's just go ahead and schedule the infusion for Thursday since I'm coming back in for the Neulasta shot (Nesta, E. coli) anyway, and that way we won't have to mess with the whole late Friday or weekend scheduling for a transfusion." (Lately, it has been difficult to schedule these procedures later in the week, with the infusion center only open so many hours.) He agreed, so I got two units of blood yesterday, which saved me a trip back today. I was still very tired last night and this morning, but this afternoon, I am quite perky with the juice of life.

I will never underestimate the importance of blood donation. A blood drive is held at my workplace two to three times per year, and a couple of weeks ago, the scheduled event drew in the largest crowd ever; dozens of coworkers each donated a unit, and many did so in my name. I am very honored by their kind gesture and know that their generosity will be a tremendous help for those people who will eventually receive the donated ju-ju.

My social calendar has been quite full recently—rather ironic, since I have been somewhat antisocial most of the year due to basically feeling like crap. The memory of how it felt to be healthy is difficult to tap, as it's been so long since I've felt normal. Even now, as I go through treatments, I am frustrated with searching for that healthy feeling and coming up empty. I do have to stop every now and then and recognize that I am going through a lot. While I have managed to stay on top of the past nagging symptoms of earlier treatment cycles, the physical and mental struggle persists. I have good days and bad; fatigue is my albatross. I want to run and jump and play and I can't. I don't know from one half day to the next how my body will feel, and it makes it difficult to plan things, although I so much want human connection. I am most thankful my family, friends, and visitors understand. I am also truly touched by how many are still reaching out to me, extending themselves to me. It never gets old. I kind of feel like Sally Field many years ago when she finally won an Oscar after several nominations and no wins and she proclaimed, "You like me, you *really* like me!" Maybe there's a Boniva commercial in my future; after all, the chemo does do some harsh things to the bones' density.

This week has been very interesting in terms of what messages the universe is sending me. It appears my last few entries have seemingly struck a chord in several people, and I am pondering the significance of the feedback I've received. I am keenly aware the impact my words can and may have on those reading my journal, and I am also aware that what I write is completely open to one's interpretation.

Above all, my intention is working through my own mental and physical healing. I am happy to hear when the words inspire and uplift, and sorry if or when they cause sorrow or guilt. I am working through so much in my brain, it sometimes literally hurts, but there is much I hold back, too private to share. I can only imagine working out all those demons and thoughts, how painful they would seem to others. I cannot write all that is on my mind—not here in this forum. I have always tried to take full and complete responsibility for my feelings and emotions. If there is mental anguish or some kind of emotional struggle in my life, I always ask myself how I can view things differently. What is my part in this pain? This has served me well and guided my moral compass, but it has also created great conflicts. Why? Because I wrongly put the expectation on others: take responsibility for your own emotions; whatever issues you have, start with yourself first. This view oftentimes shows me as dismissive and lacking empathy for someone else's pain. Sometimes people just want to vent, and I can sometimes be seen as pushing back. When overly expressed, our greatest strength can be our greatest weakness.

Betrayal and humility. I cannot think of any two more powerful or emotionally charged words, and they have been occupying my thoughts the past few days. I think of my stalwart approach to life and what I perceive as one of my greatest strengths—taking full responsibility for my feelings and emotions—and wonder how that predisposition serves during a time of betrayal. I am still trying to sort through that issue. Alas, there is a saving grace and beauty in humility. I cannot and do not have all the answers, but I ask for the wisdom and guidance to step beyond my imperfect soul to find peace in my darkest hour, when not all things seem clear. It is with great humility that I find myself here, facing this challenge in my life, and being given the chance to express, redefine, re-create, and announce how I wish to be present in this world; it is with great humility that I am supported, nurtured, and loved on this journey; and it is in humility that I wish to reside.

I Got All My Sistahs with Me

There can be no friendship without confidence,
and no confidence without integrity.

—Gaia Bistro Waitress

I am not sure if this quote belongs to the waitress at Gaia Bistro; she wrote it on the lunch bill today but did not attribute the quote to an author, so I am giving her the credit here in my journal. That restaurant has catapulted itself to one of my faves. I was there last week with my good friend Tami and went again today with my good friend and awesome hairstylist, Christiane. What I love about this place is 1) it's a breakfast place (duh), and 2) the food is organic, with many of their vegetables and herbs grown in the backyard of their restaurant or purchased locally. The dishes are divine and the atmosphere so tranquil as you enjoy your splendid meals with great company on the outdoor covered deck. Plus they write cool quotes on your bill. Love it.

I hope I never get complacent about receiving messages at the perfect time, but the above quote fit the bill. Maybe there's no perfect timing on receiving messages; maybe all we need is just a general awareness that messages are always being given—the question is, are we listening? So the quote from the waitress about friendships is a timeless one. Friendships are those unique blessings in life, and I am finding these relationships blossoming in the most beautiful of ways as I stroll through this journey of mine. I am savoring these moments I share with each of my girlfriends, as we discover more layers in each other, in ourselves.

Not only do friends keep you grounded and safe, they contribute greatly to your sense of style! The other night, I may have finally caved in about the "big bag" issue, thanks to my friend Kelley. She's got a big one. Most of my friends do. I don't. I've had the same smallish (but cute and stylish?) red purse for years. First of all, *years* may reveal my fashion *faux pas* to some of these beautiful women in my life, many of whom keep up on the trends and switch their bags out seasonally. When Ilene was here last week, I commented on her big, yellow bag. You can put small animals and dogs in these things. Clearly, I have been the holdout on the big-bag thing, until Kelley showed me the absolute utility of carrying smaller pouches within bags—little compartments of organized life all within one big fashion statement. Then I got it. See, one must appeal to my sense of style *and* utility. Now watch, as soon as I get myself outfitted with the sassiest of big bags and small pouches within, it will all be a fad and memory, and small purses will be back in again.

It's like hair; the mullet style from the eighties came back for a short time. My hairstylist, Christiane, sported one briefly just three or four years ago when she returned from one of her many trips to Germany, and she is the only person I know who could pull that off with class. I see big hair is coming back, too. That trend suits me well (of course not now, with 90 percent of my head gleaming in the sun without tresses). I had the ultimate big hair back in the late eighties and early nineties; my friends and I would perm, tease, and hairspray our locks to the highest of heights and widest of widths. Why did women have big hair? So they could hide prizes in them—this according to a *Saturday Night Live* skit from that memorable time. We thought that was hilarious, and it was our inside joke—how many prizes did we have in our hair? And whoever had the biggest hair (usually that was me) clearly had more prizes to hide!

Today, Christiane gave me this gorgeous turban wrap that she purchased for me from her latest trip overseas. She said turbans are all the rage in Europe. Those trendsetting Europeans! I absolutely love it.

See, friends keep you up-to-date and in fashion. But, while I share these stories, the point is how much these sirens add the color, the warmth, the richness to the pallet of my life. Not just in fashion, but to this unbelievable connection to the feminine spirit. That spirit, when shared with our best of friends, is so pure, so nurturing, so supportive and uplifting. It is close to divinity, as far as I can tell. There is no room for competitiveness, judgment, cat-fighting. Those feelings or actions are so foreign when true friends are gathered in confidence and integrity, as the quote above so eloquently puts it. And, as Kelley told me the other night, women should have each other's back. Not all do, but when you find those who get and understand *that*, keep them. Those friendships are precious, they are pure and worth holding on to—they are your sisters, or "sistahs," as Jackie calls them. So I raise a glass (red wine, of course, but not now because of my treatments) and toast my girlfriends—these beautiful, amazing, awe-inspiring, unique "sistahs" in my life!

Facing Mortality

It's my off week and I have been feeling pretty good overall, especially after receiving two units of blood last Thursday. Monday night was the only time I felt as if I was coming down with a cold or the flu, with some achy muscles and slight fever, but by Tuesday morning, it was gone. I have been walking again, but can't seem to shake the weight I have put on in the last couple of weeks. I feel like the Michelin Man or Pillsbury Doughboy. I went back in today for another lab draw and was a little disappointed that my platelets are down to 36 (normal range is 140 to 440), from as high as 270 just two weeks ago. The chemo really knocked those cells down. My red blood cells are in decent shape, but I thought those would be a little bit higher too, given the fact that I received a couple units of blood. I just expected my body to really rebound and produce its own blood cells. My white blood cell counts are good, since I received a shot of Nesta a few days ago. I have been having nosebleeds for several weeks now, which have been annoying. I start cycle four on Tuesday, and with this being a holiday weekend, I might have to go back in on Friday to check counts again. I want to be optimistic that my counts will rebound on their own and not deteriorate any further, but the wind got knocked out of my sails with today's results, and I am more pessimistic than usual.

Last night, Chris and I went to IntaJuice in our neighborhood to get a shot of wheat grass. Chris has been bringing me shots once or twice per week. The stuff is truly nasty. It smells awful and tastes worse. It is supposed to be very good for you. As Chris ordered, I read some of the personal notes on the wall from customers and found myself fixated on a montage of handwritten messages from employees to a particular customer. From the notes, I could tell that this particular customer died. I looked at the pictures next to the notes and saw a woman in her early forties who looked like me—bald head, puffy face. *She must have had some kind of cancer,* I thought. I looked at the top of the montage, and in big, bold letters, it read, "In Memory of Barbara." My heart stopped. I just stared at those words. How uncanny that this person also shared my name. Below the pictures was a handwritten card from Barbara herself. It was addressed to her friends at IntaJuice; it thanked them for their support and love. She wrote about how she looked forward to coming to the store to get her specific "sludge," how grateful she was that they all took the time to make this specific drink for her, and how happy she was that over time, each of the employees added their own twist to the drink. I didn't know what illness Barbara had or what she died of, but she impacted those kids' lives in such a wonderfully positive way that they paid tribute to her by creating this memorial with their own handwritten notes. The notes talked about how they missed her and wished her peace. I could feel the tears welling up in my eyes.

That incident reminded me of the story the infusion nurse told me about her first husband. Each of my blood transfusions has been administered by this same nurse, so she and I have gotten to know each other a little better with each visit. The first time I was there, she asked me about my condition, and I told her what I had. She shared with me that her first husband had non-Hodgkin's lymphoma, so she understood the battle with blood counts and chemotherapy. I didn't ask her to elaborate and concluded that she must now be remarried since she referred to him as her first husband and was currently wearing a wedding ring. *That first marriage must not have worked out,* I thought to myself. During my transfusion last week, she and I talked more. She told me her first husband died from his cancer twelve years ago. The cancer he had was fairly aggressive. He lived only one year after his first symptoms showed up and only nine months after his official diagnosis. At the time, she had a two-year-old daughter who was also having health issues. She was only working part-time, and her husband had to quit his job to focus on his treatments, so she took on a full-time position while at the same time caring for both ailing family members. I couldn't imagine what this must have been like. I found it peculiar that when she first mentioned her first husband's illness, I just assumed he lived and their marriage didn't work out. At that point, several weeks ago, most stories being told to me of people with cancer had ended positively. Several weeks later, the nurse felt more comfortable sharing, and I felt more comfortable hearing about the outcome.

Both of these stories are occupying my thoughts this evening, and I am questioning my own mortality with my current disease. Am I asking the right questions or simply burying my head in the sand? I have read and researched just enough to know that my cancer is very successfully treated. And that's as far as I've gone. I really haven't delved into other details such as complications, nor have I asked my doctor directly if I have anything to be concerned about. I am operating with just enough information to know that I should come out of this okay. But I am starting to question what I really do know, and with my counts not being where I expected them to be today, my mind starts down that slippery, negative slope. Most of the time, I am upbeat and positive, but these moments of self-doubt begin to creep into my brain. Then I start to get really down and hard on myself—am I doing everything I possibly can to ensure complete recovery? I've put on weight, and I haven't checked into yoga like I said I would. I don't always have enough energy to walk every day during my "off" week. I don't always eat healthy food. Did Barbara from IntaJuice do everything she could, only to lose her life? Did the infusion nurse's husband do everything he could, only to end up the same way? This place of self-doubt is not where I like to be, but I guess I should just allow and feel it on occasion. It is consuming my thoughts tonight, making me feel a little depressed, and I'm just too tired to fight it.

Be still and know that I am. This moment is as it should be. This, too, shall pass. Tomorrow's another day. And any other little positive saying I can tell myself to help me sleep. I will definitely need Amber tonight.

Past, Present, and Future

Today is my dad's birthday. He would have been seventy-two years old if he were alive today. He died two months before his sixty-fourth birthday. So young. That is only twenty years older than I am right now. I can't imagine having only twenty more years to live—I'm reaching for that century mark. By then, the hundreds will be the new sixties.

My father being born on this day is certainly of historic importance to my family, but what I didn't realize is it's also the same day as Martin Luther King's "I have a dream" speech forty-five years ago. Dad was twenty-seven at the time, and I was just a twinkle in his eye. I wonder what impact or impression that speech or those times in the sixties had on him. Mom was pregnant with Jeanette, their first child together. I never asked Dad about those events. I wish he were here so I could ask him now.

Today will also be the day the first African American will accept the presidential nomination of a major party. I hope that fathers and daughters and mothers and sons are talking about the significance of today's historic event so that they don't wonder later about what they each thought. Regardless of your political leanings, this is an incredible day for America. My father was a lifelong Republican; I'm an independent. I wish he were here so I could talk to him about today's events and so many other things I never asked about when he was alive. Happy birthday, Dad!

Today is also the day Chris asked me to marry him, three years ago. We had already decided to marry—weeks earlier, we had even planned our destination wedding for the following January. I had been patiently waiting for him to formally pop the question, and as the summer was drawing to a close, I was getting a little nervous, although I never let it show.

Chris's original plan was to ask me over dinner at our favorite sushi place. I had just gotten back from a business trip and was talking to him on the phone about what to do for dinner, and he suggested sushi and wondered if I wanted to meet him at our restaurant. Before I could answer, he was interrupted and told me he'd call me back. I was pretty exhausted from my business trip and really didn't want to go out, but sushi did sound good, so I called the sushi restaurant and ordered takeout that Chris could pick up on the way home. When he called me back to finalize dinner, he did his best not to show how I foiled his plan. So, on to Plan B.

Two nights later was my father's birthday. Chris and I were out shopping and he decided to pick up some filet mignons, telling me he wanted to cook me dinner. It was my father's birthday, he said, so he wanted to cook us a nice dinner in his honor. *How very sweet*, I thought. At home, he grilled up a fantastic steak and we uncorked a very nice bottle of red wine. He then asked me to tell him my favorite memories of my dad. Chris had never met my father, and he knew how special Dad was to me. He listened intently as I recalled my favorite Dad memories. Chris brought him to life for me that day.

When I paused, lingering in the memory my father, Chris reached under the dining table and brought forth a present about the size of a watch box. He said, "Since it's your dad's birthday, and he obviously can't be here to get a gift, here is one for you instead." I was so surprised, and it never dawned on me (at first) that this was a proposal. The box wasn't the right size. Suddenly I was full of anticipation, already excited over the wonderful unfolding of the evening and then this sweet gesture of a gift. Was it a watch? I tore open the wrapping and saw it was indeed a velvet *jewelry* box, beautiful sky blue in color, but it was not a ring box—it was too big—and I must admit I did momentarily think, *Why am I getting a watch, and where is my ring?* I opened the box, and centered within it was the most gorgeous ring. I gasped—this was it, this was really happening! It was a surprise, as I honestly did not expect the box I was holding to house the ring, but it did. My eyes welled up with tears, and I looked at Chris.

How perfect this day was. How beautiful that he picked my father's birthday to ask me to marry him—even if it was Plan B. Chris took this day and gave me new memories and honored our love and my father in such an amazing way. August 28 will always be a special day of remembrance for a father so loved, and of celebration for the start of a new life with my soul's mate.

✳ ✳ ✳

Great news today, as my blood counts are good! I was asked to come back today after Wednesday's counts were so low, particularly the platelet number. Today, that number nearly doubled to sixty-two. And my red blood cells are up about 10 percent, too. My body is making blood! I am supposed to have seven days off each cycle, but this time I'll only get six days off as I start cycle four on Tuesday after Labor Day.

Chris's parents fly in tomorrow. His father will be here for one week, and his mother will stay another week longer. We haven't seen Chris's dad for three months, before all of this madness started, so we look forward to the visit. Their help is greatly appreciated, especially as I start the next cycle. We have quite the social agenda lined up for the next week, with holiday weekend events and friend visits planned. I hope to be able to keep up during my treatments.

I managed to do some shopping yesterday. No big purse yet—that will be tackled at some point in the future. Bed, Bath and Beyond was my vice—that place is dangerous. My mission was simple: buy a loofah sponge to use to get rid of dead skin cells. (It was recommended to me to keep skin well hydrated and exfoliate it so that it breathes better—this helps toxins exit your body.) This simple mission netted me not just the sponge, but also a few different kitchen gadgets and a brand-new bedding set and accent pillows for our bed. I only had enough energy to power shop for an hour, and good thing, because who knows how much damage I would have done to our pocketbook. I look forward to a good weekend and feeling great and in good shape to start cycle four.

Life's Footnotes
September 2008

It is the eve of the fourth round. These twenty-one-day cycles have now become routine for me; this is my life right now, and the illness, treatments, and recovery are defining every moment. I probably have no new discoveries to unearth in terms of my body responses—at least I hope nothing negative to discover. During the past cycle, the nurse told me to expect to go through a minimum of six cycles, and likely all eight since the bone marrow is involved. She had forgotten that the bad cells were in my marrow. "That's why you're on such a roller coaster with your blood counts," she said. She continued to tell me that if the cancer wasn't in my bone marrow, six cycles might be sufficient, but definitely plan on eight. So that takes me through around mid-December. Then 2008 will be in the books. This year will be a huge black line—a demarcation—in my life. That is how I will forever compartmentalize memories and events—as life before 2008 and life after 2008.

The bone marrow is where blood and platelet cell production takes place. Talking with the nurse recently, I found out that this production takes place mainly in the long femur bones of your thighs, in your lower spine, and also in the long bones of your upper arms. While the cancer originated in my lymph nodes (hence lymphoma), bone marrow involvement makes the treatments a little tricky. The chemotherapy destroys blood cells—both good and bad cells—and at the same time I have little room in my marrow to produce my own blood as the cancer was found in both femur bones and the third lumbar bone of my spinal column, taking up space where good cell production needs to happen. I can feel that changing now. I feel the corner has been turned, and enough of the bad cells have been destroyed to allow more room for my good cells to produce. It is working.

A few weeks ago, the practice director (God himself) asked me how my legs were feeling. I told him fine, but I was a little perplexed by the question. I knew that the cancer cells showed up in the marrow of both the left and right long femur bones, and that during the diagnosis phase, they determined the cancer did not penetrate the bones, but I didn't understand why he was asking me about how my legs "felt." And I knew he wasn't referring to the muscle cramping in my quads that I had experienced after skiing earlier in the year. I pondered on this more and realized that I did have some occasional pain in the *sides* of my upper thighs over the last year. The first time I remember having this pain was the summer of 2007. I was on a business trip, and one night, I could not get to sleep because of an achy feeling in the side my right thigh. I thought it was a muscle cramp. When I was growing up, I used to get muscle cramps in my calf muscles. My sister and I both had this problem; I recall that someone told us the reason we had these pains was because of a lack of vitamin E. The only relief we would get from the pain was for someone else to massage the calf muscle or to wrap the lower leg in a heating pad. The pain sensation of those cramps was a dull ache, and that is exactly what this pain in my thigh felt like some thirty years later—a dull ache. *Lack of vitamin E,* I thought. So there I was that summer of 2007 away from home; it was nearly midnight and the pain was so great, I could not fall asleep. *I have to get some relief,* I thought. I flipped through the phone book to locate a Walgreen's close to my hotel but could find nothing. I ended up going a few blocks away to a grocery store that was open twenty-four hours, where I purchased a heating pad. Back at the hotel room, I wrapped that pad around my right thigh and was finally able to fall asleep. Then, earlier this year in April and May, there were a few nights when I couldn't sleep again because of the same pain, only this time it was in both sides of my thighs. Thankfully, I still had that heating pad from the business trip a year earlier to add to the one I already had at home. I needed to wrap both my thighs in heating pads just to get to sleep. Imagine doing this with the awful night sweats I was already experiencing.

I now look back on these moments and wonder how on earth I got through last spring without knocking down some doctor's door demanding they test me for everything under the sun. I never even told my family doctor about these leg cramps. It never dawned on me those pains were in any way connected to the host of other symptoms I was suffering from. It wasn't pain from muscles aching due to a lack of vitamin E. No, my dear, those were the cancer cells in your bone marrow squeezing out your good cells and taking away precious room needed to make good blood cells to feed your body. It is no wonder that by the time

I was tested in the emergency room on June 8, nearly one year after the first sign of thigh pain, my body had only half the blood it was supposed to have. And what a strange, long trip it has been since.

CYCLE FOUR

Breaking Spirit

Uniquely Routine

The chemotherapy session went well today, although tonight, I am feeling just a little bit labored in my breathing. My body is pumped up with so much fluid. Today, I received seven bags of "stuff." They start off each session with a bag of saline to hydrate my body. Then, as always with day one of each cycle, my blood is drawn to determine if my levels are safe enough to begin treatment. Today, they were good. As soon as I hear things are okay, I take my prednisone. Day one sucks in that regard—I have to wait to take any oral drugs until the counts come back okay, so instead of taking this happy little insomnia-inducing steroid as early as possible in the morning, on this day, I usually end up taking it about four hours later. I also take an oral anti-nausea drug at the same time. The reason for the wait is that they don't want patients to take their drugs and waste them should the treatment cycle be delayed due to low blood counts. These drugs are too expensive to waste. I received two anti-nausea drugs via the IV, then the first chemo drug, and then Benadryl to help offset the allergic reaction I get with the second chemo drug. While I was receiving the Benadryl, my chest turned red, which indicated that I was having a reaction to the first chemo drug. This had not happened before with any of the other chemo drugs except the one identified earlier, and I think it was again because the nurse administered it too quickly—it was infused into my veins in under an hour, when it should have been an hour and a half. The nurse consulted with the nurse practitioner, and they decided to give me another steroid to control that reaction—a steroid that will also add to the prednisone's side effect of insomnia. Great. This new steroid did the trick, and the rash on my chest went away, although some tightness in my chest lingered. Next was chemo drug number two, and then another smaller bag of saline, and then the third chemo drug given by the nurse through a "push," or a hypodermic needle directly into my port. I also took the oral chemo drug during all of this. Seven hours spent sitting and getting lots and lots of chemicals and fluid. My legs feel like liquid lead.

My doctor is on vacation, so the practice director sat down with me today. Our conversation left me feeling very positive about my progress. I was concerned that my heart rate has been high the past several times I've had my vitals checked, and he said that even though I am drinking four to five liters of water a day (two to three liters is recommended—I'm such an overachiever), my body may be drier than I think. He suggested drinking Gatorade as a hydrator. We talked about my low platelet count of eighty-six, and he said if I was one of his colon cancer patients, he would suspend treatment. But because I have Hodgkin's, he said that level and even lower is fine, as with this disease it is very important to stay on the scheduled cycles and the level of chemo dosage—this will improve the rate of curability. Cure? *Really?* My doctor had always referred to my illness as "very treatable, potentially curable." That word *potentially* always stuck in my brain, which sometimes sows the seeds of self-doubt I occasionally have. And here was the practice director giving me more than potential, it was a likely *probability* for a cure. I was very pleased. I then asked him when I could get a PET scan; did I have to wait for cycle six before they would recommend it? He asked me when I last had one, and I told him before all my treatments started, three months ago. He thought now was a good time to get one done and said that he would leave a note for my doctor to schedule one when he returns from vacation. I was happy with this news. I very much want to see how much of this cancer's ass I have kicked.

Chris's parents joined me for today's session. The office staff is impressed at how many different visitors accompany me to my appointments and that I am never alone. The nurse practitioner just shakes his head, giving up trying to remember the faces and names of family and friends who join me. Chris's father is a hoot. He's like my mother in that he just tells you what's on his mind or where he stands on an issue, and for the most part, he makes me laugh. Laughter is so important. Even Chris's mom joked that it looks like I'm now to wait on them, since the doctor today told us how important it is that I keep active. That made me smile.

Speaking of laughter, why do some males either leave the toilet seat up or keep the lid closed? While I enjoy my father-in-law's company, neither of these situations helps out a female with a bladder issue. It's been an adventure the past couple of days whenever I run into the bathroom—too many times at the last minute—only to find that in addition to wrestling with what should be easy-pull-down pants (everything I wear has an elastic waistband these days), I have to navigate knocking the seat down or quickly propping up the toilet lid. Of course, the same can be said from the male side of things—I am sure they are wondering why they should always have to put the seat up after us females. This male-versus-female toilet topic is nothing new, and not one I'm willing to pull the cancer patient card on, but it does make me laugh on the inside. Asking someone to change their bathroom habits just so I can avoid little accidents seems a little too diva for me.

Each cycle, I have found that the first couple days of treatment leave me a little euphoric. I am wondering if those bags of chemo drugs are laced with something to affect my mood. Or could it be my mind's coping mechanism? Whatever the reason, I am calm, at peace, and feel pleasantly relaxed during the start of my cycles. I recognized that pattern today. There is so much humility in this process that it does put me in a state of calm euphoria. Not that I am happy to be here, because this really sucks. There is that paradox again. But I am happy to have the experience of going through something really challenging, feeling the strength of my own body, mind, and spirit, and having the nurturing love and support of family and friends every step of the way. The journey one travels is so personal, so unique, but the experience of sharing one's trials and tribulations is incredibly gratifying and touching; I cannot help but be optimistic and hopeful for the future. When you understand you are not alone, you can face anything.

A Door Closing

Menopause? Excuse me? My doctor mentioned this to me for the first time yesterday, and I must admit, it wasn't something I was ready to hear. He was back from vacation and stopped in for a chat during my treatment and asked the litany of routine questions. How are you feeling? Fine. Any chills, fevers, sweats? Fevers only occasionally, but only a couple degrees. Sweats? Yes, I have been sweating some at night, not like the horrible night sweats, but I have noticed it. That could be a sign of hot flashes, he said. Then the great news: "This treatment can

bring on early menopause," he said, "especially the closer you are to fifty."
Fifty? C'mon, I'm only forty-three! Maybe he meant the closer you are
to fifty than, say, twenty. That I could understand. Regardless, I wasn't
prepared for this new information, and I am still trying to process what
it all means. I remember reading that my reproductive cycle could be
suspended (that has happened), and I vaguely remember reading that
menopausal symptoms could happen, but I didn't think the *permanent*
onset of early menopause would happen. This was very disheartening
news, and something I'm not really ready to accept as actually happening
to me. Who wants to go through menopause at forty-three?

While Chris and I have not actively tried to start a family, we also
have not tried to prevent it. We figured if it happens, it happens, and we
know we would be wonderful parents. The news from yesterday made
me sad to realize that door may now possibly be closed. I remember a
conversation with my doctor during my hospital stay in June when we
first learned of my diagnosis. Back then, he told us that the reproductive
cycle gets suspended, but in many instances, it comes back and couples
can and do conceive. So, who was this imposter doctor now telling me
about permanent menopause? I still cannot process it, nor can I really
believe it. I want to hang on to those words he told me in the hospital
months earlier.

That bit of news yesterday threw me off my game, and I forgot to
ask him about getting a PET scan after this cycle. And today, I didn't
get a chance to see the doctor, so I relayed to the nurse that the practice
director said he would leave a note with him about an earlier scan. The
nurse told me that my doctor will still likely wait until after the sixth
cycle. He normally does not do one earlier, she said.

Despite the sad news about my eggs drying up, I am feeling very
good after three days into this fourth cycle. My blood counts are in
relatively good shape. I have been working out the last couple of days
on a mini-trampoline that Chris bought me. I really had not been doing
much physical activity during actual treatment days, but this round, I
have found enough energy to get a decent cardio workout the past three
days. This morning's workout was a little harder than yesterday, as I can
feel the heaviness in my limbs, an effect from so much fluid retention,
but I am pleased my body's energy is expanding through each cycle. I
have continued to stay ahead of and control the nagging symptoms from
the first two cycles. The only thing hanging around is the weight gain

(yuck!) and fatigue. I have not been gorging myself; in fact, I am eating what I consider normal, but the steroid has a cumulative effect and is stubbornly holding on to water and extra body fat. People who visit me say I don't look like I've gained weight, but I am close to the weight I was before I started getting sick, and maybe that's why my body doesn't look any different to them. I guess the only benefit from the months of illness was the three pants sizes I lost.

We had a very entertaining evening tonight. Chris had his old work buddies over for dinner: Jeff (his ex-boss), Derek and his wife Liz, as well as Shary and Anna. We served up lasagna and chicken parmesan. Anna tried to get me drunk with her rum cake, and Chris's mom made her infamous red velvet cake. The energy level of the evening was high as stories were told and relived and we laughed loudly at and with Anna, who always manages to liven up any gathering. Chris's parents were thoroughly entertained. It was great to see Chris reunited with these old work friends; they are the salt-of-the-earth type of people and the truest of friends—ones you want around for the rest of your life.

Life's a Real Picnic

Alone. That is what I felt last night as I was watching *Stand Up To Cancer*, which was broadcast on the three major networks. It might seem very odd that I felt alone, given the love and support I feel on a daily basis, and especially based on the program's stories and statistics that showed I am very much not alone. I was alone because I was the only one watching it, by myself. Chris and his parents and I had just finished dinner, and I sat on the couch in our family room to view the show. I had mentioned the show to them, or so I thought, throughout the week, and I assumed they would join me. But, instead, they sat at the dining room table engaged in their own world, very unaware of the state I was in. And that is how it sometimes feels when you have cancer. It is a lonely disease.

The program was a fundraiser, star-studded with celebrities, and told of poignant tales of how cancer touches everyone's lives in some fashion. I am not alone, but I was sad. Maybe seeing myself as part of a statistic made it all the more real for me: 12 million people in the United States are living with a history of cancer; 1.45 million people are diagnosed each year; 19,000 will be diagnosed in Colorado this year. I am part of these numbers. The number that I am not a part of: every sixty seconds, someone in America dies from cancer. This is mind-boggling to me. That's 550,000 people each year[2]. America is one of the top industrialized countries in terms of cancer rates. Why is that? I was getting weepy from the show, so I went upstairs to finish viewing it—alone.

Patience. This is a virtue I have yet to master, one I've had very little of my entire life. It is certainly being tested now, and I don't think I'm learning well. Last night, my mother-in-law wanted to put avocado in the salad she was preparing for me. She knows I like them, but she doesn't buy them or eat them back home in Alabama and doesn't know how to peel them, but she decided to get me one yesterday. Earlier, when she asked me what I wanted in my salad, I purposely left off this item; I didn't want to bother with explaining how to select one, how to peel and cut it. There are times when I don't have enough energy to think, and yesterday was one of those days. But she bought one anyway, thinking of me, as is her nature—to think of others first. So there she was, wanting to please me with this deed, and there I was with little patience or energy to assist. And it just made for an uncomfortable exchange. If I were a bigger person, I would have just smiled and said thank you for trying. Instead, I probably made her wonder why she even bothered.

Like I said, yesterday was not a good day for me; after a few days of chemo, my moods and energy level are just unpredictable. It must be incredibly difficult to live with me during these times; my fuse is short, and I just plain don't want to think or be bothered. If you're trying to do something really nice for me, but you don't know what you're doing and eventually require my help, well, patience and kindness seem to slip from my grasp. And that is something I must work on. It's not like I had this virtue buttoned up before I got sick; it's always been a struggle for me. Ask my husband. And my mother-in-law. Or to be fair, any one of my siblings who grew up with me. So, go ahead and throw in chemotherapy and the possible onset of early menopause, and I am sure these low-energy days of mine are a real picnic to be around.

I went to bed last night determined not to wake up in this same cranky state and with low energy. I don't like being there. (Let's face

---

2   *Stand Up To Cancer*, television program, directed by Louis J. Horvitz (2008, Los Angeles, CA, Entertainment Industry Foundation).

it; I don't like being *here*, sick.) That determination paid off as I awoke feeling better, and the first thing I did this morning was work out on my little trampoline. And one of the springs broke. This is the second one this week that has broken—no, not because of my weight gain, but because this particular trampoline was constructed poorly. Chris was determined to get me one (he is very pleased to see me physically active), so we stopped at REI after breakfast—nothing there. Finally, at home I researched mini-tramps on the Internet, found a good-quality one—of course with the price tag to match—and ordered it. I can't wait for it to arrive, because I have enjoyed my morning bouncing. So, today is turning out fabulously, my energy level is great, and I am trying to keep active.

Later this morning, I received an e-mail from my friends Kim, Christin, and Liz—all three wonderful friends from book club who have since moved from Denver to San Francisco, Washington, DC, and Boston, respectively. The three of them got together and hired a personal chef to cook a few meals for me one day this month. How very exciting. (What was that feeling of being alone and cranky yesterday? Seems so far away.)

Chris dragged me to Costco this afternoon—"To keep you active," he said. He also wanted to show me that they had a Vita-Mix blender on sale for a limited time. This mixer is something we've considered purchasing for months, and Costco had a great price, so we picked one up. A necessary start to our journey of healthy food and juicing! And tonight, my family is coming over for dinner. Right now, my mom is here with my mother-in-law, and they are preparing pot roast and vegetables for all before everyone else arrives. The aroma in my house is delectable and so incredibly comforting because my moms are cooking it. And this is how my roller-coaster life is these days: the ups and downs, alone and not alone, the low and high energy, the impatience and patience, but always the hope for healthier days, always surrounded by love, always seeking a different way to view life than in the saddest of my moments, always knowing I am going to be okay and always being grateful for the humility of it all.

Bittersweet

The whoopie pie. That scrumptious dessert defined my childhood and that of my siblings. What is a whoopie pie, you ask? It is two devil's food chocolate cake cookies with a marshmallow cream center. Think Suzy Q, but so much better and not so "processed." This is an east coast treat that my mother perfected when we were growing up back in Maine and New York, and she brought her infamous recipe here to Colorado, but over the years, lost it. Many attempts were made to find a substitute recipe; even my sister made this treat a few years ago from a recipe she found on the Internet, but each attempt was met with disappointment. I have dreamed of one day tasting this sweet delight, but wondered if the taste and memories would ever cross my palate again. Until last night. Brother Michael called to tell me he was running late for dinner because he was making a surprise. And what a surprise this was! While he didn't make the exact version, it was 95 percent there, and I have to say, life is pretty much complete now that this dessert has been resurrected again in our households. I held the chocolate-cake-like cookie in my hands and breathed in the aroma of dark chocolate, my mind flooded with childhood memories, as I took a bite into the decadent bliss, the cream center squishing into my mouth. The look on my face must have been priceless, because my brother beamed with pride and said that reaction was just what he was looking for.

Michael's sharing this experience with me and the family last evening was all the more poignant, because today, he could have lost his life. I was at my sister's tonight celebrating my nephew's eighteenth birthday when she told us Michael wouldn't be coming. He had notified her earlier in the afternoon via phone text that he had an accident with his bike and was getting stitches—that was all it said. I did not like the sound of the cryptic message, so I called him to get the details and found out that the incident was much worse than any one of us could have imagined. Michael has taken up extreme downhill mountain biking, and this afternoon, he crashed hard on the mountainside and was knocked unconscious for a couple of minutes after cracking his helmet. That cracked helmet could have been his skull. He is resting fine, finally home late this evening after a few hours in a mountain-resort emergency room getting stitches to his nose, upper lip, and a gash in his hand and having a splint put on his left thumb, which is probably broken. He has multiple bruises and road rash, having taken part of the mountain with him. He told me that someone who saw him crash just watched his body go limp after he hit the ground. I can't even begin to process the information that my brother could have lost his life today—I cannot fathom another crisis happening in this family right now. Thankfully, Michael was very alert when we spoke and in good spirits. Rick is going to stay with him this evening; he suffered a concussion, and the ER doc advised that someone stay with him overnight and wake him every couple of hours. I so want to help out, to be the sister to go to him, and I can't. I hate it. Our family is running on fumes right now.

I came home from my sister's house and hugged my husband hard, then went and ate a whoopie pie. It didn't taste as sweet as the one I had last night.

Cancer's a Bitch

I'm under house arrest again. My white blood cells are almost nonexistent at .4! I have to stay away from the general public, away from sick people and anyone exposed to sick people, and avoid eating raw fruit and vegetables.

My doctor was AWOL again, so I spoke with the practice director (herein referred to as PD). These two have varying viewpoints on treatment. Both agree with the aggressiveness of the chemotherapy treatment, which is good, but they differ on their approach to care. According to one of the nurses, the PD is more likely to order up more scans than some insurance companies require, while my doctor is more traditional and will wait until after the usual six-cycle count for my type of cancer. Thus, I am not counting on getting the PET scan after this fourth cycle, as I was so excited about last week. The PD told me today that with my white blood cell counts so extremely low, if my fever were to spike to 100.5, that would mean an automatic hospital admission for me to receive antibiotics intravenously. I have a feeling my doctor would say, "Call me and we'll talk about your other symptoms, which, if you have none, take two Tylenol and go to bed." So far tonight, my temperature is holding fine around 97 degrees (although I am getting hot flashes, which could be due to that wonderful onset of potentially permanent menopause—fabulous).

My other counts today were okay. My red blood cell count actually held up well over the last few days; the shot of gerbil ovaries from Thursday probably helped. I got another rodent shot today. Platelets are low at 37, crashing from the 80s of last week. I am hoping for a post-chemo-treatment bounce (sorry, can't seem to avoid the political lingo). I go back in tomorrow for Nesta (E. coli) to boost those white blood cells. And then I am back in on Friday for another blood check, and, heck, if I need a transfusion of platelets or red blood cells, I'll certainly take it, but with my recent good energy days, I am feeling my body rejuvenating itself. After today, no more chemo drugs (except my not-so-good friend prednisone through next Monday).

Chris went out of town today. He has been working hard on a proposal he's presenting at the home office in Philadelphia tomorrow, and I wish him well. Actually, he should kick ass, because that's what he does. He's been burning the candle at both ends, which has had the unfortunate effect of interrupting my sleep the past couple of nights, but with the two of us in separate states tonight, we should get caught up on our z's. His mother is here through Saturday. I am working on that patience thing and finding that I do better on the days I am less challenged with fatigue and depression.

By the way, remember when I wondered if the chemo drugs from days one through three had something laced in them? Well, I asked the nurse today about my feelings of euphoria, and she confirmed that yes, one of the intravenous nausea drugs is a steroid, and one of its side effects is a state of euphoria. She also told me that you can have a letdown a couple of days later. How true! On Friday of last week, I felt tired and slightly depressed. Well, today, I received this happy steroid again and must admit I am feeling a little high, but fatigue is trying to knock on my door. (Stay away!) Decradon is the name of that steroid. I think I'll honor that one steroid on my list of BFFs with the first male name, Derek. Derek, in honor of Chris's old work buddy and our good friend. And how fitting—Derek gives us all a nice, euphoric feeling whenever he's around (and especially with a Pabst Blue Ribbon or Natural Light in hand).

I spoke with Michael today. He is doing better, although still quite banged up. My sister visited with him yesterday and says she was taken aback by the facial trauma he endured; she says he looks like he was in a really bad fight and lost. My poor, sweet brother. I hate hearing about the pain he is in. He managed to get himself to his family doctor, who looked him over and determined that he didn't need any further x-rays or treatments, even though he complained of neck pain. The only thing the family doctor told him to come back for was to remove his stitches from his chin and lip on Friday. Michael has an appointment with a surgeon tomorrow, the one specialist the emergency doctor already knew he needed; he broke his left thumb and has a large gash in his palm. He is wearing a splint dressed by the ER doc and will likely get the area re-set with a cast. I know Michael already feels bad for having some family attention diverted from me to him, but he needs to get over it. Life happens at us, and we stick together, no matter what. I only wish I could be there for him like he has been here for me. I had planned to visit him tomorrow, but with my house-arrest status, I am disappointed I won't be able to, and that sucks. Cancer's a bitch.

One Human Race

Today is September 11. Several years later, it is still difficult to escape this date without some reflection of those tragic events from 2001. I was at work when a coworker turned to me and said that a small plane just crashed into one of the World Trade Center towers. *That's weird,* I thought. Then, what seemed no longer than a few minutes later, he announced to me that a second plane did the same. And that's when you knew something was horribly wrong. Some of my friends and family witnessed on live TV that second plane ripping a hole into the second building, a gaping exposure of humankind's ideological wars. Such a gut-wrenching, soul-searching, incomprehensible time in our collective history and memories.

I don't know if this is the same for anyone else, but for me, just the appearance or utterance of the numbers nine and eleven together is a constant reminder of that painful day. Several times during the course of a week, I will see those numbers, usually when looking at a digital clock. I am simply checking the time, as I often do throughout the day, and for some reason I catch myself looking at the clock when it reads 9:11, either in the morning on the bottom right side of my computer screen or at night when contemplating bedtime. I probably glance at the time of day a hundred times during my waking hours, but the digits 9:11 have a meaning unlike any other number combination. (Maybe December 7, 1941, had a similar hold on the American psyche—the day that will live in infamy—but there were no digital clocks back then, and once the rawness of the event had time to pass, no subliminal daily reminders, just the anniversary date.) I stop and pause each time I see those numbers. It's as if the universe wants me always to remember and never forget. I wonder if others have that observation, or if it's just me.

There are two things I remember most about that time surrounding 9/11. One was getting violently ill one morning a few days later. My body just gave out over the horrific senselessness of it all and I was puking my guts out—I called in sick that day. But what I also remember is the incredible strength and unity of the human spirit, which connected us to each other in a way like nothing else I have experienced. (Something close to the experience of this unified spirit came after the tragic event of the Columbine shootings here in Colorado in April 1999. I remember walking through the memorial-dense forest of cards and posters hung in the park next to the high school and seeing a glimpse of the world crying for us.) No matter what our beliefs and differences, we lost a part of our souls that day, and in the days and weeks that followed, a new part of our universal soul was born—one that was stronger, more resilient, more loving. History shows it often takes tragedy to remind us of our true humanity. Seven years later, while it is prudent for us to remember and never forget, we collectively—and sadly—have managed to slip back into our old routine, are involved once again in our selfish beliefs and political bickering. It should not take a tragedy to remind us that we are all one human race. Can we get there without these jarring events?

I sit here writing about this and think of my own internal struggle with my disease. I continue to contemplate what it all means, still search for purpose, and frankly just find myself exhausted from the exercise. I have the complete desire, drive, and responsibility to myself and to my loved ones to heal. Today I am tired, again, trying to find the energy to tell my body to rid itself from any of those stubborn, lingering cancer cells and rebuild fresh new blood cells. It is a constant physical and emotional battle. Always, I have to remind myself of my blessings. Always, I have to turn my thoughts to the positive. I am halfway there. This thing is almost kicked. I feel it. But the days are hard, and I am so tired. I cannot wait to feel normal again, to grow my hair, to run and sing and dance, to touch others' lives, to have purpose, to spread love, and to remind everyone we are one human race.

Restless Exhaustion

Well, I couldn't get through this cycle without some much-needed juice. I had definitely been feeling my body crash since Tuesday of this week, and by Friday, my blood counts had confirmed what I was feeling. I had always thought that the exhaustion is mainly due to a low red blood cell count, but the nurse told me that combined with an extremely low white blood cell count, fatigue is even more exasperated. I had no idea. My white blood cells continue to be near nonexistent, but should be rebounding even as I write this, as it's been about three days since getting the shot Nesta, and it takes a couple of days for efficacy. After getting a unit of platelets (my count was at a new low of 7.45) and a unit of blood yesterday, I went back in this morning for a second unit of blood. I haven't been able to work out for a few days due to the fatigue, but tonight, I am finally getting some energy back. I am looking forward to several days on the rebound before the assault starts again.

The randomness of it all is something I am trying to get my arms around. I asked my doctor last week if there was anything I could read in the patterns of my counts that would indicate how far they will go down, or stay steady, or rebound. For example, my platelets did not crash during cycle one, but did during cycle two. During cycle three, my body significantly produced its own (being given an extra week off due to my infected biopsy site), maintained a higher level, but then crashed to lower numbers than cycle one. My platelet count was at a higher level beginning with cycle four than both cycles one and two, yet here I am crashed to the lowest number yet. My doctor told me there is nothing you can point to that would show an exact pattern or a proportional relationship of how the chemo tears down the good cells. It is frustrating, to be sure.

The fatigue I feel while my body is crashing is almost debilitating. I don't know quite how to describe it. Despite my exhausted state, I can't just go to sleep and then wake up refreshed. That feeling isn't afforded me; the only thing I get refreshed from is the infusion of blood. This persistent fatigue is chronic and restless at the same time. My sleep is constantly interrupted during these crashing days, despite the fact that all my body craves is sleep. Even on Amber, I am sleeping lightly, waking up every couple of hours. REM sleep does not exist during these days. I am zombie-like, lifeless, short-fused, easily irritated. I am no fun to be around. I don't even like to be around me. It's like being a "Mini-Me" inside your full-sized body, and you want to jump up to see the world through the eyes of your old self, but you can't reach them, so you are trapped in a shell that's bigger than what you can fill. What's worse is I don't have the energy to explain this to anyone while I'm experiencing it, and so it is difficult for others to know how to communicate with me or help me—and thus, understand me. Trying even harder to be accommodating or overly attentive to me only makes it worse—it's too much stimulation. What I want is to scream that this sucks and throw a tantrum—kick my feet and pound my fists—but even a release such as this escapes me; there just is no energy. And so I just veg, exist, hang out, until my body reaches its low point and I am granted the juice of life. I need the blood; I want the blood. It is the only thing I can count on during these days to get "Mini-Me" to grow back to my full-sized body.

Saturday nights during my recovery have been spent with my family, but tonight, it's just me and Chris. His mother went home today after her two-week stay. (It probably felt like a prison sentence to her.) My sister and brother-in-law are taking their kids to an anime event this weekend. Rick and Ron have plans with friends, and Michael has to work (and is also doing well recovering from his accident). So, it's me and my hubby, and we are delighted to be spending some "us" time together. After we took Chris's mom to the airport, we went to see the movie *Burn After Reading*. A great flick. I was in tears laughing so hard by the end of the movie. Beware, though, it is a dark comedy, and the Coen brothers do not disappoint.

It was an absolutely gorgeous day today, barely a cloud in the sky, a perfect temperature in the seventies, the sun shining so intensely and warm, a cool breeze telling us fall is in the air, and portending cold winter days ahead. And I am juiced up, regaining my energy, and spending this beautiful day with the love of my life. Life is good.

Cue the Angels

With last week's platelet and blood transfusions, I've had a couple of great energy days until today. I woke up very tired, not sure why. I haven't been getting good sleep for several days now, and maybe it's catching up with me.

On Sunday, Chris and I went to the gym. I hadn't been there since the middle of May. I had been reluctant to go, not just because of my weakened physical state, but because I look so different now. It's obvious I'm sick, and to be at the gym with a bunch of healthy people just wasn't a motivator for me. Even so, I managed well with about thirty minutes of a workout on the treadmill. The last time I was at the gym in May, I could only do ten minutes of exercise on the elliptical machine and had to stop to rest every minute. This was because I was so anemic, although I didn't know it at the time. On Monday, I worked out on my new mini-trampoline that finally arrived last week. (I didn't break it this time, either—a much better-quality unit than the ones we had previously purchased.) So, two good days of being physically active, and then today hits and I just feel run-down. I'm not sure if I'm trying to fight a cold or what, but some of my muscles are just a little achy, I have a headache, and my nose feels as if it's getting stuffy. I've been eating a lot of sugar and sweets lately—dessert about every day, sometimes twice per day—and my weight is reflecting it. I feel like such a slob. Yuck.

Today, I also had blood checked, and while both my white and red blood cell counts have rebounded from last week's growth shot and transfusions, my platelet count continues to be challenged. I'm at 19 right now, up from 7.4 on Friday. I am not sure why my body is not making more platelets. If I'm this low on Thursday when they draw blood again, I'll likely need another transfusion. Infused platelets do not last that long, just a few days. *Produce, body, produce!* My white blood cell count is good at 11.6, but the count is usually much higher after Nesta, so I'm a little concerned that I don't have quite the buffer I'll need going into the next cycle. My red blood cells are okay, but I did expect them to be slightly higher too. If the numbers trend down even slightly, I will ask them to give me a unit of blood. I just don't want to start the next cycle in a lower state.

Chris went out of town today and will be back Thursday night. I have been alone and on my own all day, the first time I have not had someone with me at least part of the day. When I went in for my blood draw, the lab tech even commented, "Are you alone? You are never alone!" And she's right; I have always had someone accompany me to all of my doctor appointments. So, I am a little depressed, not because I'm alone, but because I've been looking forward to being able to exercise my own independence. Being tired during my off week even one day seems so unfair. Maybe I tried to do too much the last two days, or maybe it's the change of the season. I get so few great days when I'm not getting chemo; it truly sucks to feel so off, especially after being so active yesterday. My looks, the weight, the sluggishness; I'm really just getting tired of this whole thing. I was supposed to go to a friend's house for dinner but just don't feel up to it. I'm in such a funk.

On a couple of different occasions last week, I ran into people who I had met early on in this journey. One of them, Laura, the young twenty-six-year-old girl who has been battling her illness half of her life, was in the doctor's office one day last week. I hadn't seen her for more than two months, and we had a chance to catch up. She recently volunteered for an organization that provides companion care for senior citizens. Her assignment is to a lady who also happens to be blind. Laura visits with her companion periodically to take her on outings, or she just sits and keeps her company. Here is this girl, this angel who I referred to earlier in my journal, dealing with her own disease and finding time to extend herself to another.

The other person I saw was the ER nurse who was instrumental in setting my recovery path in motion. Last Friday, Chris and I were in the waiting room at the Sky Ridge infusion unit when we saw this nurse, Kathy was her name, and we waved at her. She smiled and said, "Hello, my friends. How are you?" Then she disappeared behind the double doors into the ER. It has been more than three months since that fateful night of my initial diagnosis, and it surprised me that she had even a glimmer of recognition for us. In those three months, how many shifts and how many new patients must she have seen? And I no longer look like a frail, anemic waif with long, brown hair. I was sure she wouldn't remember the circumstances. Moments later when I was sitting in the transfusion room, hooked up to an IV and waiting for the unit of platelets, Kathy walked in to greet us. "I wanted to come find you and see how you are doing. Please, do tell me your names again."

Kathy is in her forties, petite, blonde, and English. I reintroduced myself and Chris and briefly told her what has transpired since that night in the ER, my official diagnosis and treatment plan. She leaned up against the wall and crouched down next to Chris to have a more intimate conversation with the two of us. She clearly remembered that night with us and even recalled all the family members that had come to see me later in the evening. She really cared. And she saved my life that night. The ER doctor was ready to send me home that evening back in June, and it was Kathy who insisted my blood be checked for anemia. The doctor obliged, and the rest is history. She never took credit, even though we kept giving it to her—she still referred to it as a total team effort. I thanked her again for her thoroughness and insight that night, and as I spoke these words, my eyes welled up with tears. I couldn't believe how emotional I still was, even three months later, but this woman with her genuine caring spirit was the reason I finally got some answers to the months of my ill health. She smiled and thanked us for being so kind.

On days like today, when I want to bury myself under my covers and not come up for air, all I need to do is focus on these two beautiful souls with giant hearts and a giving nature, who inspire me and have touched me in such a way that I cannot stay down for too long.

Social Addiction

As much as I hate the way prednisone makes me feel during my treatment and how truly elated I am when I finish each cycle's dosage, going off of it during non-treatment days crashes me hard. That is what I determined happened to me on Tuesday. I went off the happy steroid that day, and I suffered the effects of withdrawal. I didn't recognize it at the time, but I do recall that during cycle two, I had a similar reaction: body crashed, fatigue, achy muscles, and headache. I talked to my sister today and mentioned this to her, and she said that when she has had to administer this steroid to her children (in much smaller dosages), the dosage instructions from her pediatrician start low, increase over a period of days, and then decrease again. Makes sense. And here I am taking a very high dosage for fourteen days and then quitting cold turkey. I'll need to remember that day fifteen of each cycle could be a down day for me. Thankfully, yesterday and today have been good days.

I had my blood drawn again today with good results. White blood cells are in normal range, down a little bit. My hemoglobin (part of the red blood cell count) jumped to 11.5—I think that is the highest it's been since I've started treatments (a normal range is 12–16)—and hematocrit (also part of the red blood cell count) is at 33.6 (normal range starts at 36). I have noticed from past transfusions that a unit of blood seems to increase the hematocrit number by three basis points, so my body has produced the equivalent of about a unit of transfused red blood cells in only two days. Yay! My platelets are up, but still at a low count of 28. I am producing, but I really need to get that number higher, and I expect it be higher when I resume treatments next Tuesday.

Speaking of treatments, I came up with this brilliant idea of "chemo dates." Through each of my cycles, I have not been alone on chemo days in the doctor's office; I have always been accompanied either by Chris or a family member, and on occasion an out-of-town friend. Next week, I start cycle five. Chris has no travel plans and will be home working, but I won't be requesting his presence during this cycle. This will be the first time I will be going to and from appointments alone, and I have decided to ask friends to visit me for a couple of hours on each of my long treatment days next week, which I am calling "chemo dates." Since it has been a running joke with some of the office staff about how many different people have accompanied me during treatments, I think it'll be hilarious to have two to three different visitors throughout the day—keep 'em on their toes.

I have always thought of myself as quiet and reflective, and one who relishes time alone. Ironically, it is through this journey that I am recognizing how much I crave social interaction with my siblings and good friends, and of course, my husband, just as much as I want my space. Before I got sick, I used to plan for alone time or "me" time, a chance to reset my mental compass. Now, I find myself planning for social events, and it is this connection that I need for mental balance. I am alone in my thoughts all day. Alone time is available to me at any moment; all I have to do is go upstairs to my retreat. And here is the beauty of my Web page: it is my social connection to the outside world. And as much as many have told me how great my Web site has been as a communication tool for them, it has been like a lifeline for me. It is interesting how attached I have become to this tool, and how I am moved by the posts that are written, and how depressed I can get when no one has posted for days. A post is like being tucked in for bed each night; the comfort of knowing someone is thinking of me, someone is caressing my head, someone is blessing my soul is like a drug. Each post is like getting high, and each day without a post, I go through a kind of withdrawal. It is the oddest thing watching myself go through these emotions.

A friend who survived Hodgkin's twenty years ago told me several weeks ago that this will happen: soon, friends stop checking in on you, they get back to their lives and you don't hear from them; then all you can rely on is your family. Internally, I dismissed her experience, figuring that she was just a teenager when she went through her challenge, so of course her emotions and perspective would be different than mine.

I know what she's talking about now and understand those feelings are real. It's no one's fault; it is just life. There is not one person who cares about me any less than they did two weeks ago, two months ago. Life goes on for everyone, and I must never forget how grateful I am for each soul who has blessed my life in some way.

Acceptance. Add that to patience, and I see I still have much to work on.

A Medical Emergency

I lost my dignity last night around 6:30. I was lying on a bed in the ER room at Sky Ridge (why, I'll explain later), when my lower abdomen started to twist and cramp and I knew I had to run to the bathroom. The only problem was that the shared bathroom attached to my room was occupied. I cried out to Chris, "I have to go!" Chris knocked on the bathroom door, and finally a toilet flushed. *Whew,* I thought, *I am barely going to make it.* The lady's voice inside said she was finished, and Chris heard her leave through the bathroom door attached to her room on the other side. Unfortunately, she failed to unlock our door from the inside of the bathroom. Chris pounded his fist loudly on the door, hoping the lady could hear him from her room—she didn't. *Oh my God,* I thought. I started to get nauseous, and my entire body broke out in sweats. I curled up on the bed in a fetal position, rocking and moaning, and screaming out to Chris, "I have to go *noooooowwwwwwww!*" Calm, cool, and collected, Chris grabbed a small, pink washbasin sitting on the counter. It would have to do. I stood up and ripped off my hospital gown because I was so hot, Chris put the plastic washbasin on the floor, I squatted over it naked, and out flushed the bloody diarrhea—the reason for my being in the ER room. I fell back on the bed, ready to pass out, covered my body with my gown and whispered to Chris to get help. Stench filled the room; the basin still sat on the floor next to my bed, holding the proof of my latest ailment, when in walked a half dozen of the ER staff ready to assist. The ER doctor introduced himself and instructed the nurse to get an IV set up immediately. And just like that, I went from being an ER patient who was calmly waiting for blood results to a priority case, having almost passed out from my condition, the proof in the pink washbasin, plus a putrid smell permeating the air and penetrating everyone's nostrils. I had no more dignity at that point.

It all started late Friday afternoon. It had already been a wonderful day as I spent a few hours watching the personal chef hired by three of my BOTS girlfriends prepare a week's worth of gourmet meals in my kitchen. After she left, Chris and I sampled one of her scrumptious meals. Chris then retreated to his office, and I suddenly felt tired and found myself dozing on the couch. I awoke, still quite groggy, and went upstairs to check my e-mails. I suddenly felt the onset of pressure in my lower abdomen and ran to the bathroom. I went diarrhea, saw fresh, dark blood on the toilet tissue, and panicked. I sat down on my chaise and called for Chris. My heart was racing, and I started to get nauseous with anxiety. I was freaking out because I knew this meant I was bleeding somewhere internally, and with my platelets so low, this was not a good thing. Ten minutes later, I had to go again, and this time I looked in the toilet—it was completely red with blood. I called my doctor's answering service—twice—and after no return call in almost an hour, Chris and I decided to go to the emergency room. My mind thought the worst: where was I bleeding? How would they stop it—surgery? Wouldn't that be dangerous with my platelets so low? Finally, the on-call doctor called back and I explained to her what had happened, where my last counts were at, and that we were on our way to the ER. She agreed with our decision, although I will say she was much calmer than I was. As I was getting my vitals checked at the ER, my heart rate was 130 beats per minute. The nurse's aide asked me why it was so high, and I told her because I was worried about bleeding to death.

After my public display of diarrhea in the ER, the nurse got fluids flowing into me and I started to feel better minutes later. My blood count results came back and showed that platelets were up from yesterday's 28 to 47, so that was good, but red blood cells had decreased, indicating I was losing blood. I was wheeled to radiology for a CT scan of my abdomen. They were checking for anything acute, such as tumors or colitis. The results came back normal. Whew. After a couple of hours, I was moved to the intensive care unit, where they transfused a unit of platelets and two units of blood, as well as lots of saline solution and an antacid drug that would also aid in healing my digestive tract. I had never been in intensive care before. Basically, I was hooked up to every monitoring device imaginable so the staff could keep an eye on all my vital signs. I was told I could not have anything to eat or drink until I met with a gastroenterologist in the morning.

Chris stayed with me overnight, and we both got a few hours of sleep off and on. In the morning, I awoke feeling better than the night before, and since I hadn't had another bowel movement, it appeared the bleeding had slowed or stopped. This morning, we also met with the gastroenterologist. He suspected I might have an ulcer, particularly since I am taking such a high dosage of naproxen daily. He said he recommended at least an endoscopy, which is a test of the upper gastrointestinal tract. If he found an ulcer there, he would cauterize it (burn it). But, if all was normal, he would then schedule me for a colonoscopy for the next day, Sunday morning.

The results of the endoscopy were normal, so now I am scheduled for the colonoscopy tomorrow. I can finally have liquids, but nothing to eat except popsicles or Jell-O. Starting at 5:00 tonight, I will drink four liters of a liquid that is supposed to clean out my lower intestines so they can have a better view during the procedure—this means more diarrhea. We shall see how that colonoscopy turns out; I am hoping it is nothing more than a burst blood vessel or polyp.

The Waiting Game

It's Monday morning and I'm still in the hospital, waiting for yet another procedure. It was supposed to happen at 9:00 AM, but as 9:00 AM rolled around, they told me it is now scheduled for 1:00 PM. This procedure is called enteroclysis, which is a special x-ray of the small intestine— something about a tube through the nose and contrast liquid and lots of x-rays and pictures taken of the small bowel area. Joy. I was completely frustrated to find out the procedure was changed, because I am starving. I've had only one solid meal since Friday afternoon, and that was dinner last night. Other than this one solid meal, I have been ordered to have either no food at all or only a liquid diet of broth and popsicles and Jell-O. I guess this is one way for me to lose some of that prednisone-induced weight.

Very little information has come so far, and that, too, has been frustrating. Even the colonoscopy procedure I had yesterday was delayed from the morning until 3:00 pm—another frustration. Those results showed I have five ulcers, which the gastro doc biopsied. Results from the biopsies could take days. The doctor did not talk to me after the procedure, as I was still recovering from the anesthesia, but he spoke briefly to Chris. He asked him if the cancer I was being treated for was detected in the colon, and Chris told him no. Chris said he didn't really tell him much more after that, so of course I assume the very worst and wonder if the doctor thought those ulcers were cancerous.

So, after yesterday's experience and this morning's delay and having very little food the last couple of days, I reached my breaking point and just started crying. I called my oncologist's office because I knew my doctor would take charge and help me understand what was going on, only to find out he is on vacation (*again?*) until next week. The receptionist told me they would send Jay, the nurse practitioner, to see me. I hung up the phone and more tears flowed. I'd just about had it.

When Jay arrived, he told me he didn't think the ulcers were from the chemo I was receiving. He thought what was going on with me was "odd," and that they (gastro guys and radiology) would do everything they could to figure out the cause. Until then, he said, chemo is suspended, for at least a week. Physically, I feel fine. I have had three units of blood transfused since Friday night, and the blood count results every four to six hours have continued to show stabilization. Jay said he told the hospital staff to extend the blood count to every twelve hours, as it seems I am doing well. Even so, before he left, he told me I could be in the hospital for one to two more days. Aaaargghhhh!

Thankfully, not everything is so dreary. I was moved to a regular hospital room last night, which, after two days in intensive care, was a blessing. I didn't think I belonged there; patients on that floor were truly very sick. When I arrived in my new room last night, one of the nurses who tended to me during my last hospital stay in June was on duty. She walked into my room with a big smile on her face and gave us a warm welcome. She said she saw my name on the patient list but I had been assigned to another nurse, so she asked that nurse to trade with her. I was so moved that she remembered me and wanted to be assigned to care for me. Then this morning, one of the nurse's aides who had also cared for me in June stopped by to see how I was doing. That hospital stay in June is a time I will never forget, since so much of my life was in tumult and about to change. What I will always remember is how wonderful the staff was to me and Chris while we were here. To be here again more than three months later and have these incredibly sweet and caring women not only remember us but be excited to see us—it's just something that warms my heart and helps dry my tears of frustration.

Home Sweet Home

I was finally discharged from the hospital on Tuesday. They actually could have released me early evening on Monday after my last procedure, but there was no doctor on the floor to sign the discharge papers and I had to wait until yesterday afternoon before a doctor was available to see me. As much as I have raved about the services at Sky Ridge, I am mostly referring to the accommodations and the care from the nurses and nurse's aides; as far as relying on any of the doctors, forget about it. Trying to get any time or answers from the myriad of doctors who had some hand in my treatment and stay was frustrating to say the least. This is probably the case at any hospital, I would imagine.

These past few days have really rocked my world and Chris's. We have spent most of today in downtime, just trying to recoup from the incredible inconvenience of my latest health issue. Luckily, nothing acute or abnormal was discovered in any of the tests conducted, and no definite conclusion could be drawn on what caused the bleeding. Speculation is that either one of the discovered ulcers bled or possibly some small, undetectable fissure bled. And with platelets so low, the blood oozed and pooled in my lower intestines and was expelled as disgusting, bloody diarrhea until my platelet-challenged body could finally clot on its own and heal. By then, I had lost quite a bit of blood. The unit of platelets and three units of blood helped, and by the time I left, my body was producing its own blood, raising my counts even more. I was physically exhausted, mostly from little sleep and restlessness and the procedures, but I knew overall I felt okay and that my body was fairly strong. And on the positive side, it was good to get my entire digestive system scoped; I would probably not have had any of these procedures done at this point in my life were it not for the problem.

It was interesting looking at the pictures from the endoscopy and the colonoscopy—it surprised me to see how "clean" and pink the insides look. Both of these procedures were relatively painless, and with both I was sedated and given that drug that gives you amnesia. Unfortunately, I was not sedated for the final procedure on Monday, the enteroclysis. That is because this procedure requires the patient be alert in order to receive instructions from the radiologist. It was awful! Having a tube shoved up my nose and then threaded down my throat into my stomach and small intestines was the most uncomfortable I have been in any medical procedure, ever. As if that wasn't enough, a wire was then shoved through the tube, air was pumped into my stomach, and then nearly two liters of liquid was injected through the tube. Every two minutes, the radiologist kept asking if I was okay, and no, I wasn't, but I was a captive with nowhere to go. Give me chemo any day, but please don't put me through that procedure again.

The other inconvenience of these past few days has been the delay in my chemo treatments, which has screwed up the "chemo dates" I had set up with friends this week. I was so looking forward to social time with my friends who graciously arranged their schedules to spend time with me. Cycle five would have started yesterday, and now no chemo is scheduled until I meet with my oncologist, who seems to have more vacation days than office days. He is back next week Tuesday, and it's possible he will have me come in the very next day to start treatment, but I won't know for sure until then. And I can't really reschedule chemo dates on that kind of short notice. I'll have to wait until cycle six to allow my "dates" to plan accordingly. Bummer.

So, it's nice to be home. Chris and I spent today relaxing and trying to get life back to some sort of normalcy. As much as my body is put through, mentally and physically, I must not forget how much this impacts my husband as well. He slept on a reclining chair all four nights at the hospital, ate horrible food, and basically was there for me every step of the way. It was a good thing he wasn't traveling. And now I realize and understand his concern about leaving me alone and his insistence that someone be with me when he is gone. I can no longer argue the point, and I must say my confidence in my own rate of recovery has been knocked down a couple of pegs.

Last night was nirvana, sleeping in our bed and falling asleep in my husband's arms.

A Silent Prayer

It is hard to believe I was in the hospital just a few days ago. With great blood counts from Friday and a good weekend, I am feeling pretty close to normal. Cancer, schmancer. I think I'm healed. I really think they should just give me that PET scan. I'll put that on my list of questions for my always-vacationing doctor. I meet with him on Tuesday afternoon. I won't have an official start date for my next chemo cycle until my doctor reviews with me the latest episode in my health journey, but I am expecting he will schedule me to start treatment the following day, Wednesday.

A week and a half ago, I was on top of the world, ready to drive myself to treatments and have social chemo dates with my girlfriends, and then my body betrayed me with internal hemorrhaging. That whole episode really knocked the wind out of my confident sails, set me off course and out of balance. I looked ahead to this upcoming week and potential treatment days and began to plan who of my family could watch over me, knowing Chris would have to refocus himself on work. But today, I am back, and I think I may be able to drive myself to treatments this week and manage just fine. All I needed was a couple of days to process the events and sift through the negative thoughts invading my once-impenetrable bubble of confidence. My body felt strong after I left the hospital, and my energy built with each day; so, too, did my belief in this body to heal itself. The great counts on Friday only confirmed this mounting surge of strength, and I rewarded myself with a relaxing pedicure, the first I have had since being diagnosed. This morning, my family was over for a delicious brunch. Tonight, our masseuse was here to massage away all the hospital-stay stress. Last weekend: bleeding, blood transfusions, ICU, little sleep, no food, and horrible procedures. This weekend: relaxation, yummy food, pedicures, and massages. Oh, what a difference a few days make!

It has been a challenging week for my family. My mother was very concerned about me, as were all my siblings and my in-laws. My sister has been especially challenged, as just last week, her husband was diagnosed with multiple sclerosis (MS), a degenerative autoimmune disease, which he'll battle for the remainder of his life. I was very saddened to hear this news. I understand the physical and mental struggle of facing a disease, the label of no longer being healthy, of being less than normal. It seems so unfair. But I also know the blessing of having incredible love and support from family and friends, of finding an inner strength that I always knew existed but the depths of which I was unaware of until now, and am still uncovering. The opportunity for self-reflection and discovering what life is really all about, what's really important, are such incredible gifts that I don't know that I would trade this crappy cancer for what I have experienced in terms of personal growth. I still have so much to learn, and yet I'm convinced I would not have taken the time to delve this deep, to recognize beauty in places I never looked, to hear and feel the promise of eternal love and life in the whisper of the wind or in a child's laughter. It is not easy, but that's what makes the journey worthwhile and the lessons that much more meaningful.

I pray that my brother-in-law will find his own inner strength to see past the pain and incredible inconvenience of having a disease that he didn't ask for. I hope he finds the beauty and love that life offers us. I pray for my sister, who now worries about not just her sister's well-being but her husband's as well. She may feel very challenged and overwhelmed, but maybe she doesn't recognize her own strength and the healing power that her love bestows on those of us close to her. I pray for both of them and hope they find new ways to appreciate each other, just as Chris and I have done. I pray for strength for my family that we never forget to extend ourselves in love and support for one another, in the manner that my father taught us.

CYCLE FIVE

Balancing Act

The Rush of Fall
October 2008

I'm back on the chemo wagon, just completed day one of cycle five. I drove myself to and from the doctor's office—a first for my chemo days. Michael came down to sit with me for the day, and we had a great time hanging out. We both had our laptops open, and I surfed the Net and kept up on all the interesting news stories going on currently in our country. I have been a news whore of late, oftentimes flipping between all the cable news channels while also scanning for the latest economic and political stories on the Internet. Treatment went well today and was uneventful, very routine at this point.

I absolutely love this time of the year—fall. Today, I am enjoying the beautiful fall weather these days bring us: wonderfully radiant, warm days and brilliant fall colors with cool evenings. The fall also rushes in new beginnings: football and the start of school. Football will forever be a special link to my father. As the quintessential Daddy's little girl, I got many cues of what my future interests would be by observing my father's interests. I probably wasn't much more than four years old when I jumped up on the sofa and sat next to my dad while he was watching football. "Who do you want to win, Daddy—the guys in the purple or the guys in the white?" It was one of my earliest childhood memories, and my love for football was born on that day. I also always looked forward to starting school. I loved learning new stuff and seeing all my friends after a long summer off.

Some people don't like fall because it spells the end of hot summer days and freedom and the cool nights foreshadow a cold, dreary winter. But the year-round intense warmth of the Colorado sun and the deep blue sky with nary a cloud in it, anchored by the majestic Rocky Mountains, are more than enough to keep these negative views at bay. Oh, and the colors this time of year—the crisp yellows and golds, the fiery reds, the brilliant oranges—are such a feast for the eyes. There is nothing that can diminish the beauty this time of year brings to my soul, not even a round of chemo treatments, nor this intrusive disease.

Maturity and Grace

Tonight, I am tired. I did pretty well today, day three of my treatments. In fact, the past three days have been okay, but it's catching up with me now. Fatigue. Bloatedness. I am pregnant with gas. Same old, same old. It's all becoming so routine and so tiresome. My counts from today were pretty steady eddy; in fact, my white blood cell and platelet counts were up. Even my red blood cells were in good shape this morning, down only slightly from a couple of days ago. But as the hours tick away, I know the chemo is breaking me down. I feel it. Today's visit was at the doctor's second location on Hampden, and they rushed me through my treatment because the office closed early with staff meetings scheduled for the nurses. Even so, I didn't have my usual allergic reaction, which was a good thing.

My brother-in-law, Ken, joined me today for my treatment. Ken has been part of our family for more than twenty years, and this is the first time I have ever spent this much alone time with him. And it was long overdue. Neither of us would say that we have had the closest relationship in those years; much of it had been filled with the immaturity of youth and egos. We would both agree we are glad those days are behind us as we have aged—not so gracefully, at times—into two mature individuals, more comfortable and accepting in our in-law-relationship skin. And now our relationship is taking a unique twist and we are connecting on another level because we are both chronically sick. Ken has been battling physical ailments off and on for ten years. Some earlier testing years ago pointed in the direction of MS, but nothing was definitive. Recently, he has been suffering more intense symptoms, which prompted more testing and finally the confirming diagnosis of MS last week.

We had a great talk today, sharing our fears, our struggles, our hopes, our desires as we face illness. He was very kind to me in his compliments of how I am handling my health challenge, and he wanted to draw on that strength and inspiration. I was humbled by his words of admiration. He said that I have somehow touched his soul, and that is the most satisfying of compliments I could have received. I hope I was able to offer him some insight, assure him of his own inner strength, yet validate the very real struggle he faces. Our time together was a blessing, a reminder of the importance of family, love, and acceptance.

My sister, his wife, is our link. She has been the loving beacon of light that has soothed us both in our times of need. Together, Ken and Jeanette have raised beautiful children with good hearts and good intentions. I know there will be tough times ahead for Ken, but there will also be new discoveries and opportunities for deeper reflection on life and its meaning and prioritizing what is important. There is no challenge too great that love cannot overcome.

The Promise of Equilibrium

Gloom and doom. There's uncertainty and uneasiness all around. Just turn on the TV, read the newspaper headlines and, Henny Penny, the sky is falling. I admit I am too entranced by the news of the day, and usually I can exercise control over the remote and do something constructive to keep my mind off the negative stories. But this time is different. It seems the pervasiveness of our economic and political problems is compounding, affecting the globe; it is hard to ignore. And this backdrop against fighting cancer is all the more troubling. I don't like it; it is upsetting. I am not worried about my healthy recovery because that, I am sure, is certain. But I am unsure about my own finances, even though Chris and I are fiscally responsible, frugal, and well disciplined with our own economic house. Still, it is a scary time in our lives watching the nation's economy collapse, and it is difficult to pull away from the drama. No one is without blame, I feel, in a world where we are all connected in some way. It is a pivotal time in human history, and it will be interesting to see how we humans show up and sort it all out. Chris is concerned about how all the outside news is impacting me, but as I explained to him, I need to feel what I feel, and in the end, I have the utmost faith in the universe balancing itself out, as it is attempting to do now.

And I have proof in this balance. As this energy has been pulling me down of late, today I received a nice package that instantly changed my mood. A friend of a friend sent me a gift accompanied by a nicely written letter; her words were of comfort and support for my struggle and a sincere thank you for how I have touched her life by the sharing of my journey. I call her a friend of a friend, but I have known her for years, mostly as an acquaintance, but as someone I have admired and respected from afar. Turns out, she has felt the same way about me, and she shared that with me in her letter.

It seems the word *friend* is redefined for me on a daily basis, and for the most part, what I am uncovering is the sheer and utter joy and genuineness in such connections. I've mentioned on a couple of occasions how a couple of close friends have seemingly stayed on the sidelines, and even though I have tried my best not to be affected by my own preconceived notions or judge the behavior in any way, at times, I'm not that successful. What I am most grateful for is the strengthening of many other friendships and the promise of a deeper connection with newer friends on the horizon. I cannot wait to be better so I can be fully engaged in these new relationships.

During my extra time off last week, I shared breakfast (of course) on separate occasions with two wonderful women, each of them friends of friends or family and more than mere acquaintances to me. I have always admired these two women and felt a warm connection to them. One I've known for about five years, the other more than a dozen, and this was the first time I have spent alone time with either of them. It is this illness, this disease, that has opened up the opportunity for greater relationships. Or perhaps it is the willingness to bare my soul, to expose my vulnerability with honest expression, that has opened up a path of light for our souls to connect. I only hope I can honor these new friendships with the same meaning and beauty of spirit they have shown me. They are the reason I have faith in this world. They inspire me, and they are helping me heal.

Love, Pure and Simple

Mom came with me to chemo treatments for the first time today. I had been somewhat protecting her, not wanting to inconvenience her with sitting for hours in an uncomfortable chair with her portable oxygen tank. In doing so, I may have been inadvertently excluding her from my experience, and that certainly was not my intention. She has been very worried about me, as any mother would be for her child, and the internal hemorrhaging from a couple of weeks ago so scared her, she was shaking when Rick told her. My mom. My sweet, sweet mom. I so love and adore her.

Last week, I decided it was time to have her over again to stay the night and spend some good quality time with her and bring her to one of my chemotherapy sessions so she could meet the people who are tending to my care. Today was a good day for this, as day eight of my treatment cycles is the shortest—about two hours in the doctor's office. My mom is certainly more than willing to endure the long hours of my chemo sessions, not to mention all the ups and downs of my roller-coaster journey. One of my biggest challenges is allowing those who love me to make the decision of how they want to help me, and accepting that what I may view as inconvenience for them, they may view as an opportunity to help. My mother would do anything for me, and I stop her from what I view as her limitations. This, I think, is my way of showing how I care for her, but I must be careful not to insult or diminish her desire to show how much she loves me.

She is one feisty woman; the debates over our varying viewpoints on today's current economic and political environment—views that over the years have only hardened and continue to keep us entrenched on opposite sides—have been colorful and animated, to say the least. I love my mom for all her convictions and principles, no matter how they differ from mine. And at the end of the day, none of these varying viewpoints holds a candle to the strength of a mother's bond to her child. There is nothing more comforting than a mother's love.

My blood counts were very encouraging today. After seven days of treatment, my counts are higher than they've been at this point in time during previous cycles and almost as high as when I have started each cycle. This is very good news and tells me that I have significantly more room in my bone marrow to manufacture my own blood cells; it is no longer being crowded out by the cancer cells. Having the extra week off from the internal-bleeding episode seems to have helped my overall recovery, despite the doctor's insistence that aggressive twenty-one-day cycles be the norm. I imagine they would not want more than a week's delay for any reason, and that has happened twice already. Even so, I feel stronger; I feel that I am healing.

And I have been thinking about when to return to work. I feel guilty on the good days, thinking I should be trying to figure out a plan to be more productive. I am challenged, as these days are still somewhat unpredictable, and unfortunately, that unpredictability does not lend itself to contributing to work on a consistent level. Chemotherapy in general, and the treatment I am on in particular, is a bitch. It is devastatingly hard on the body. I'm feeling better, but it's all relative. Even though I finally had a couple of days before this current cycle where I felt better than I had this entire year, the chemo starts all over again, poisoning my veins and providing the ultimate paradox of this journey: tear down the body before it can heal.

I had an interesting encounter today while at my doctor's office receiving treatment. The woman sitting next to me was receiving chemotherapy for colon cancer and we struck up a conversation. She is cancer-free, yet in her fifth year of treatment. I was perplexed. Why was she here if she is cancer-free? She explained to me she is on a maintenance program. She had stage IV colon cancer, and while it was eradicated within six months of diagnosis, the seriousness of the disease and the likelihood of recurrence are high enough in her particular case, and frightening enough to her, that for the last five years, she has been coming in each month for three days of chemotherapy as a preventative measure. She is not yet fifty years old and actually looks younger. The treatments didn't seem to be tearing her down outwardly. She told me she went on short-term disability during the intense therapy in the beginning, and that after becoming cancer-free, she returned to work but continued the regimen of chemo-maintenance. Over time, she received less support from her employer in allowing her time off for treatments. At the time of her diagnosis, she had been with her company ten years (*same as me*, I thought), and three years after she returned to work, she finally quit her job under the mounting pressure and lack of support from her employer. She said she had been the insurance provider in her family, and when she quit, she switched to her husband's lesser policy. Then, earlier this year, her husband was laid off, and she has been on COBRA ever since to maintain the same coverage. Her husband finally got a new job recently, but they have a ninety-day waiting period before she can join his new insurance, which, unfortunately, provides even lesser benefits than his previous plan. The guilt she shared with me about wishing she were more productive upon returning to work and now not being able to be the contributor she had been, coupled with her husband's layoff and lessening insurance coverage, all hit too close to home for me. Don't get me wrong—I am lucky and blessed. I have a highly treatable and potentially curable disease; I am employed and on short-term disability; my husband has a wonderful job related to a strong industry (oil and gas). But these are scary days, as I have said, and the tether of rope between what I have today and what this lady sitting next to me has is thin and taut, especially in today's economic environment.

My husband, bless his heart, is the calming presence of light in the psychological tug-of-war my brain plays with me. Even though I have this faith of balance in the universe, I still have creeping doubts about the unknown, and it is his vision that is clearer and his confidence that is stronger. He is my rock. He sticks by me no matter what I think, no matter how I physically feel, no matter how different I look—his love knows no bounds. A mother's love and a husband's love. I am a very, very lucky girl.

The Fishbowl Effect

Despite the great counts last week in the middle of my cycle, I definitely felt the crash of my body last Thursday, Friday, and Saturday. It appears that my roughest times are days nine, ten, and eleven of each cycle when I need to have blood transfusions. But no transfusions were ordered this time, and I probably could have used a unit of red blood cells to perk me up through these couple of days. Finally, this morning, I awoke to find that my head was no longer in a fog and my body no longer dragging in exhausted fatigue. That tells me that possibly the eight days of chemo drugs have worked their way through my body, so that now, on day twelve, I am starting to regroup; maybe the blood-cell breakdown has stopped and my body is finally winning the blood-production war.

And just in time, because today I went to the Broncos game, a big outing for me, considering the energy output necessary when attending a sporting event. The past three days of fatigue had me worried that I may have to cancel at the last minute, but off to the game we went. It is amazing how simple outings such as these are not so simple when you are ill. Chris and I were guests of his business associate, who for the last few years has taken us to at least one Denver Broncos game per year. I have always looked forward to these events, being a big football fan (although a fair-weather Broncos fan). Usually, we meet up for lunch prior to the game and hike up to the stadium, take our seats, drink beer and cheer and sneer at the game's unfolding.

Today, I was a little challenged and slow in getting around. It was cold, drizzling rain at times, which hampered the experience somewhat, but I managed to stay comfortable. I did take notice of my surroundings in a different way, however. I felt like I was in a fishbowl most of the game, observing the fans around me, the play on the field, the lights and scoreboard, even the rain, and somehow felt I was separate from it all. I was watching this game as a person with cancer. Generally, I have not been too self-conscious about my condition when out in public, but I did feel different today. Alone. Apart. Separate. On occasion, I was involved in the game, getting riled up and yelling out at good and bad plays, cheering and aw-ing with the crowd around me. But for the most part, I was cocooned, hiding under layers of clothes, trying to be incognito.

At one point, I looked around and for a moment felt an appreciation for the testosterone pulsing around me. There were plenty of women fans, to be sure, but they were far outnumbered by their male counterparts, as is typical at major sporting events, and it was the men I noticed. I marveled at their bellicose enthusiasm, their sheer joy for the game, for being in this moment in time with their buddies, drinking beer and howling loudly and with such affirmative approval as bodies on the field slammed into each other at full speed. There was something so primal about it, and I found myself silently honoring the ritual of being male, the bonding and sharing of the masculine, connecting each of them without words spoken, yet clearly understood by the men around me. It was at that moment when one of the younger male specimens, who had been fully engaged in his being male all game long, turned around to me and said, "You have to be the most adorable thing in a blue rain poncho that I've ever seen." It made me smile. Heck, it made my day. Okay, he was young, clearly inebriated, but somewhere, somehow, in this bubbling masculine soup, he must have sensed my self-consciousness, my separateness, my aloneness. Chris then leaned over to me and said with a sheepish grin, "Did that guy just hit on you?" And in an instant, I was pulled back to reality, no sensing males here, noticing my silent plight. Just a bunch of happy, carefree guys having a good time. It was as simple as that. And that simplicity made me smile even more.

＊　＊　＊

I give up trying to second-guess this whole blood thing. It's my off week, and I haven't been able to string together two good days like I typically can at this point in my cycle. Sunday was a good day—went to the game but paid for it dearly on Monday, when I was tired most of the day, unable to do much activity at all. Tuesday was a better day, and so was today until this afternoon, when after lunch I started to feel fatigue set in again.

The visit to my doctor's office confirmed lower blood counts. I'm right at the point where I could decide to forgo the Procrit shot or even a blood transfusion and trust my body to make up the difference, but with only a few more days until the next cycle begins, I decided to go ahead with the quickest way to perk me up, and that is blood in my veins, now. Tomorrow, I will go in for the juice, two units. At first I was disappointed that I seemingly have not been able to maintain and sustain my own production, but then I reminded myself that I have received five units of blood: two at the end of the last cycle and three during my impromptu internal hemorrhage. Those units were infused less than thirty days ago, and thirty days is about how long transfused blood lasts. So it makes sense that those cells are beginning to expire and my own production isn't enough to make it up.

Such is the ongoing battle. That's okay. It has to be. I will write more tomorrow when I am hooked up to the IV. I'm tired right now and need some shut-eye.

Spitting Nails

I am grumpy and irritable. This whole illness thing is getting on my very last nerve. I hate feeling this way and bitching and moaning about it, but I am sooooo over it. I want to be done, to be healthy. I am getting cynical and crabby.

I was at the doctor's office and hospital yesterday for more than three hours. What should have been a routine blood draw and doctor chat was drawn out to what seemed like eternity. I spent maybe twenty minutes total discussing my current issues with a doctor, nurse, or hospital employee, but it took more than *two hundred* minutes to get those precious twenty minutes of discussion. Our health care system is for the birds. Hurry up and wait.

One huge source of my frustration has been waiting on the results from the colonoscopy done almost four weeks ago during my latest hospital stay. They told me when I was released from the hospital to call the GI doctor's office if I hadn't heard anything after two weeks. I did, and after several phone calls and missed messages, it took one week to discover that his office did not have the lab results because there was no release form signed in my file at the hospital. Why they didn't have this release form already, having performed two other procedures on me in the hospital where they did give me results, is apparently irrelevant. I signed another release form last Friday and as of Wednesday, still had heard nothing. Yesterday, since I was already visiting my oncologist, I went down to the medical records office at the hospital to get this information. When the administrator looked in my file, she told me that there were instructions given to the lab to send out results to all doctors attached to my case: the gastroenterologist, my oncologist and family doc. Yet the lab sent results only to my family doctor—the one doctor least involved with my case. Aaarrghhh! In a system driven entirely by process and procedure, the patient is relegated to the background and incredibly inconvenienced. There is no such thing as customer service for the patient. It doesn't exist. It is so difficult trying to keep your medical affairs in order when you have to constantly be vigilant about your treatment and managing your information, particularly when you are feeling like shit. Where is the patient advocacy? My cynicism says it doesn't exist.

I hate this hole that I am in, and I want to crawl out of it. Chris says it's better than the alternative. I presume he means death and, of course, logically he is right. But logic is not what I want to hear right now. This sucks. And anyone going through battling a disease and trying to make their way through the quagmire of our health care system understands what I am talking about it. I hate the way I feel, the way I look, the utter sense of a loss of control. The very experience and the accompanying negative thoughts are dangerous and have the effect of pulling you down further into the abyss. It is a vicious cycle. Juxtapose this against our country's current economic malaise, and I just want to spit nails and tear out my hair (the last three remaining strands, that is) and just rip out of my very skin.

"Snap out of it!" Isn't that what Cher declared as her character slapped Nicolas Cage's character across the face after he proclaimed his love for her in the movie *Moonstruck*? That is what I find myself doing on a daily basis, sometimes multiple times a day. There are battles on many fronts: mental, physical, and universal, really. The fields are all interconnected and enmeshed, reliant on a steady grasp of reality. Should any front fail, surely the others are unavoidably impacted. And of course, the same is true if they are positive and succeed. Aaarghhh, stop this roller-coaster ride—I want to get off!

Alrighty, then. There it is. I am done bitching. Whew, feel better.

I am currently at the hospital, getting infused with that nectar of life, packed red blood cells. It is my friend. I am a little doped up on Benadryl and sleepy. I know what is on the other side of this: energy, a lift in spirits, and a wide grin on my face. I have one important full-time job, and that is recovery. More than one year of feeling crappy and four months of aggressive tear-your-body-down treatments are not insurmountable. I will do this. I am doing this. Chris is right; there is no alternative.

Mental Thrashing

I am back, thank goodness. The past week, which was supposed to be my off week, was difficult, even though I had a couple of good days. It wasn't just the fatigue that plagued me (as is always a culprit), but the mental depression was particularly acute. There was a lot of stuff heaped up on my brain, and I really struggled with maintaining a positive outlook and drowned myself in negative thoughts, mostly aimed at disgust with myself.

The seeds of this self-betrayal were probably sown a couple of months ago. As I looked ahead in my recovery back in the summer, I pegged this timeframe, around mid-October, to have some goals set, attained, and surpassed. I thought I would be feeling better physically and able to put some kind of health regimen in place that would involve healthier eating, yoga, or some kind of physical workout routine. I also thought by this time I would have set a goal for myself on work; I thought I would have known by now if I was able to start back to work at least part-time, or have a date in mind when to return. I thought I would have a game plan for investigating a writing career on the side.

I have arrived at this point in time—the future which is now the present—when I figured all these goals would be realized, and not *one* of them has been. And I feel I have let myself down completely. It's not that I'm lazy, although my brain tried to hold that against me, too. That hemorrhaging episode really took its toll on me and my progress, setting me back a bit. And, as my doctor also explained last week, as I was so exasperated at having low blood counts during my off week, the chemo has a cumulative effect over cycles, rendering any effort to stick to plans a crap shoot.

Thursday and Friday were particularly difficult, as I could only look at myself in the mirror and wonder, *Who is this stranger?* The body—twenty-five pounds heavier, pasty and white and bald, puffy face, arms, neck, and a gut that enters a room long before I do—is foreign. I was disgusted, depressed, even angry. How does my husband look at me and even want to stay with me? I didn't want to talk to anyone and I didn't want to go out much, although I managed just a couple of outings with friends when my energy level was good. I couldn't see a light at the end of this miserable tunnel. I curled up with my laptop and blogged with people on various political Web sites and spewed my venom at them instead. *Anything to avoid dealing with me.* It was a vicious, vicious cycle I found myself in, and physically I couldn't fight back, I was so tired.

Finally, late yesterday afternoon, the clouds began to part, the fog lifted from my brain, and the transfused blood from Thursday was beginning to inject energy and some much-needed positive thoughts into my brain. My sense of control that had been an occasional visitor this past week was finally ready to move in for good (at least a few days before the next cycle). Now that my clear-mindedness has arrived, I've got to figure out how to stay ahead of these negative emotions and the mental thrashing I do to myself when I am physically crashing. At least now I've experienced the mental dark side, and I hope I am able to recognize the signs before I drown in misery again (and without the necessity of medication).

It is Saturday and I am sitting on my back patio, watching my husband do yard work with his shirt off. It is amazingly warm, almost eighty degrees, the sun's rays hugging us both as we go about our tasks. A few weeks ago, we added seven trees to our backyard, and Chris is now moving dirt and rock around shaping the landscape, his body glistening against the Crayola-blue sky on this absolutely gorgeous autumn day. A cool breeze glides through the yard like silk, taking with it a few crumpled brown leaves loosely hanging from the ash tree's branches. I close my eyes and take a deep breath, ushering into my soul the smell of grass, dirt, and sweat. I am here in the present, so grateful for life. I am back and so alive.

A Call Answered

Dear Vicki,

I was thinking about you today, like I do just about every day. And I was wishing I could get some advice from you, like you were so good at and so willing to give when you were with us. Chris and I were talking today, a rather serious talk. He's been concerned about my focus on getting healthy, as he's noticed how depressed I had been the past few days, and wonders why I don't reach out to people in my same condition or seek out a support group. I told him it's not in my nature—asking for help—and I always try to solve things on my own, spending a great deal of time internalizing my situation and mulling things over in my head until I can find my own strength, which usually always leads to action and solutions. He's been frustrated with me because a) he says he feels what I feel—if I am depressed, it brings him down, and b) he is a man of action and a man who knows how to use resources, and when confronted with an issue or challenge, he instinctively goes about finding a solution, rather than dwelling. He sees me dwelling. But I'm not; I am just internalizing.

Anyway, the point is, I don't see the usefulness of seeking out strangers in a support group for me—I feel the fight with cancer is such an individualized journey, everyone's situation is uniquely his or her own. But if you were here, I would be sitting down at your desk and asking for your advice. Because you went through your own battle with cancer and because you know me (and Chris, for that matter). But life isn't always fair, and you are missed more than you know.

As I watched you go through your very personal struggle with breast cancer, I remember marveling at your incredible spirit and positive attitude and how you were so willing to share your story with any of us who asked. I only wish I would have spent more time with you, and I wish I would have asked more about what you were going through. Who knew that as you were so bravely fighting your battle, cancer was waging a war within my body?

It was your optimism and love of life that kept all of us hopeful that you would beat this thing. When you went into remission, there was little doubt in anyone's mind that you had the upper hand. And how devastated we all were to learn the cancer had returned after several months, and with a vengeance. It was fast, Vicki, for all of us. And when I saw you in the office this past December, I really didn't think that day would be the last time I'd see you.

Ironically, it was at that time when the silent cancer in my body had secretly gathered enough strength that it was starting to show up symptomatically and I was beginning to lose weight and feel much fatigue. Over the next several weeks and months, I remember checking in with others at work on how you were doing, and always the news was that you were hanging in there, feeling good, alert, and full of love and life and spirit. My heart went out to you, and at the same time, I was getting worse; not knowing at all what was ailing me, not once thinking I was plagued with cancer.

It was a very tragic day this past spring when I heard of your passing. I called a colleague of ours to give him the sad news and found myself breaking down as I was leaving the voice mail, the sober reality hitting me only as I spoke the words that you had lost your fight. And it was just a few weeks later that cancer in my body was no longer silent as I learned of my own diagnosis. I have thought of you every day since. I wish you could advise me now, Vicki. Not some stranger.

As a young manager over the past few years, I had sought your advice and counsel on numerous topics, from employee issues to developing my own management style. Always, you were available to listen and always with the utmost respect and impartiality. You shared your knowledge and wisdom on matters from legal to personal. I never once left your desk feeling like I wasn't heard, even if the answers weren't easy. Chris felt the same way, and we often commented on how we valued and trusted the professional relationship we had with you. Somehow, you made professional and business feel personal and comforting. It is this comfort I seek now.

And tonight, you answered that call. It was during my massage therapy session this evening that I found my mind focusing on you, and I found my soul wishing you were around. The masseuse was steadily manipulating the stress and toxins from my muscles, helping me relax. Then she put her left hand on top of my head and placed her right hand on the small of my back and held that position for a moment. While she kept the one hand steady on my head, she slowly moved the other hand to different points on my back (chakra points, she later told me), holding each position for a minute or so. I started to feel a calming energy transferring from her palms to my body, comforting me. *And then you were there.* I was lying facedown on the massage table, but in my mind, it was you I saw standing over me, and it was your warm hands placed on my head and the middle of my back. You were smiling, and in that moment, I felt the incredible nurturing touch of a mother, a friend, a wise soul. It was as if you were saying, "I am here." All the doubts, negative thoughts, and sadness were released from my tired body. I felt so light, so relaxed, like warm liquid poured onto the massage table. I was at peace. So much so that I was overcome with emotion and tears flowed.

Thank you for visiting me, Vicki, and comforting my soul. It was just what I needed.

With love,
Barb

CYCLE SIX

Being Human

The Sweet Scent of Horseshit

Friendships have a way of expanding and enriching your world, and this illness of mine is allowing me time to know my friends in a deeper and more meaningful way. And as I've written here many times before, I am thoroughly enjoying this part of my journey. I love uncovering these different layers, learning the unique qualities of each of these beautiful souls whom I am so blessed to have in my life.

This week marked the start of cycle six and the long-awaited "chemo dates." Yesterday was day one, and I spent time with two friends at the doctor's office and had another friend come by and share dinner she had prepared for me. (Rick was here last night as well to stay the night since Chris was out of town.) Today, I had two more friends sit with me during my treatments, and tomorrow I will spend time with another friend.

These friendships are truly like fine wine: they indeed get better with age, their color intensifies, their scent (essence) unfolds like a gorgeous bouquet, their taste (how it makes your soul feel) is smooth as silk, and the more you drink in their beauty, the more you appreciate the complexity of every sip. We are aging gracefully, my friends and me. Each of us feeling more and more comfortable in our own individual skin, each of us experiencing similar events on one level, and different events on many other levels, but all experiences blending together to make a whole, unique gift of a person. We offer this gift to each other with an open heart and a full appreciation and respect of our familiar traits and our diversity. I love my friends.

As I get to know them, it never ceases to amaze me the new things I find out about them. For example, my dear friend and hair stylist, Christiane, unveiled something I didn't know about her—a new hobby she has discovered that is truly unique, so different than what I imagined her doing. But as she described this new joy of hers, the passion with which she spoke brought it to life right there in my doctor's office as chemo was coursing through my veins and made me forget where I was because for a few minutes I was right there with her in the middle of an open field riding a horse and *herding cattle*! That's right, this is her newfound love, and it makes her heart sing. My hair stylist—who is a walking fashion plate, so gorgeous and tall and beautifully German, with eyes that sparkle green and beam a light straight to your heart when you have her undivided attention, who pairs a sassy pair of jeans with any top and smart pair of fashion boots and does not shy away from any color—she walks in a room and you are immediately drawn to her. Now, this description (quite accurate, I might add) would make her blush, because I know she does not believe she draws such attention, as she is at first a bit introverted around strangers, but believe me, she does draw you in. She knows hair, she knows style, and she is very good at what she does, which is why I go to her, and why my white, shining, bald head cannot wait to start sprouting hair so she can do her magic and make me feel whole and beautiful again. But vanity aside, the real reason I've entrusted her with my mane is because she is my very good friend with a huge heart and her worldly experiences and rich points of view enhance my life. And here she was yesterday visiting with me at my doctor's office, and she reveals to me this new side to her, this desire she has had for the out-of-doors and being on a dude ranch or farm. She actually told me she loves the scent of it all, even the cow- and horseshit. Seriously! *Gawd, how can anyone not be entranced by this person?* I thought. So honest, so bold, so brave to admit such a thing.

Cancer took her mother's life two years ago, and I remember the heart-wrenching updates in the e-mails she sent to us from Germany, as she cared for her mother in her final days in her home country, helping her transcend from this life to the next. On each anniversary of her mother's death, Christiane has decided to honor this time and cleanse her own mind and soul by getting away from it all, preferably in the great outdoors so she can be one with nature and the universe. Unbeknownst to me, she had an interest in the farm life and animals. I was equally in the dark about her love of horses. Christiane explained to me that she longed to go back to a particular dude ranch she had visited within the last year, but when she found out it was booked and unavailable, she set about finding another similar experience. When she came across cattle herding, she signed up.

She spoke of her adventure with such color and life: basically herd eighty female pregnant cows to the winter pasture and keep them away from the country highway, which is where the cows would expect to be directed to get to their usual pasture. (In the past, the country highway had been closed off.) But this time, she explained, they were told to herd the cows to a different pasture, and that the herders would meet some resistance. Cow revolt! I marveled at her story as she told of scary moments when some cows got too close to the highway, which was not closed. Christiane had to gallop ahead of them and urge them to change direction. This took some time before the heifers were finally convinced of the new path they were to take. I learned about how the cows, over time, will pick their own "leader" cow and instinctively follow this leader's actions.

"As a herder," Christiane explained, her green eyes latched on to mine, "you must convince this leader of the new direction, and the others will eventually follow."

"The herd mentality!" I exclaimed, so engrossed in her story.

She told me how much she learned from the wranglers (guide instructors, if you will—one of them was a lesbian dairy farmer, a story within itself). I loved listening to Christiane and mostly learning about how brave and bold my dear friend was for following her heart and jumping into life. And all of this brought forth in celebration and honor of her mother's life. She so enjoyed this adventure and discovered a parallel life she can lead without impacting the current one she lives and also loves. She will participate in an upcoming two-day herding and then partake again next year when the cows are brought down to spring pasture. A new radiance glowed from her beautiful face, her eyes were dancing with joy, and her soul was literally singing—I could hear it. She inspired me to examine my own passions more closely and follow what makes me happy.

This is the beauty of true friendships and the unpredictable gifts they bring you; inspiring tales of acts of bravery and bold follow-your-dreams stories, which usually come when you least expect them but most need them. Just make sure you are listening and ready to receive, because they may come in the form of farm animals and horseshit.

A Common Thread

Chris and I voted yesterday. It was the first time I have ever "early" voted. Election Day falls on my off week, but I figured I would try to get this very important task out of the way instead of braving the potential long lines on that day. It's easier for me to gauge how I feel *at the moment*, rather than predict how I'll feel in a few days. I spent yesterday morning poring over the state amendment ballot issues, and when we went to our polling location, there was no line, and it took just a few minutes. It felt good to cast our votes and do our part to participate in the American electoral process. We have so much to be thankful for in our democracy, and the freedom to cast a ballot, have choice, and be counted is a privilege and right we should never take for granted.

Speaking of things not to take for granted, I continue to receive well-wishes and greetings from complete strangers. My aunts in Pennsylvania have put the word out to their respective Bible and church groups, and over the past months and most recently the past few days, I have received wonderful letters of encouragement and support. I also continue to hear from Chris's family and their social and church friends as well, the same sincere and genuine letters of hope and blessings. It touches me deeply to see communities come together in prayer for me, a stranger, out of the pure love of their hearts and commitment and belief in their faith and God's ability to heal. I feel the healing power of their faith.

Interestingly, both Chris and I have strong Southern Baptist ties in our families, yet neither of us practices this faith, nor do we belong to a religious denomination. We both have a humble appreciation for the diversity of faiths that all our family and friends practice or believe. The common thread through all the messages I receive from them is of love, kindness, faith, and healing—a big bear hug from the heavens and the universe itself. All these positive thoughts coagulate and converge into one safety net underneath my feet, and I feel safe and supported; fears and weariness evaporate. Months into my journey, I am still receiving these well-wishes, reminding me that I am not forsaken.

I am in day five of cycle six and feeling good, taking it easy. This past week, a couple of nurses commented that this may be my last cycle—a change in their position from several weeks ago when I was half-heartedly pushing for an early PET scan at the completion of cycle four. Back then, they dashed my premature hope to beat this thing in record time, short of the eight cycles they were preparing me for, but now they are changing their tune a little bit. I am trying not to get too excited about it and am taking their comments with a grain of salt. I am scheduled to have a PET scan week after next at the conclusion of cycle six. I am encouraged and cautiously optimistic that I will have positive results in my progress against this disease. It is just a matter of time before I will declare that I am cancer-free, I know it.

Earlier in the week, a dear friend gave me a bracelet, a circle of words etched in silver, words that so appropriately have great meaning to me now: *Happy. Cherish. Connect. Honesty. Love. Goal. Virtue. Relax. Respect. Believe. Giving. Peace. Dream. Heart.* I will wear this bracelet and draw on the energy from these powerful words and the well-wishes from friends, family, and even strangers, to never forget the opportunity of life this journey is showing me.

Circle of Life

House arrest again. My white blood cell count is at that *dangerously* low level again, basically nonexistent at .7. Today is day eight of chemo. I went in expecting both white blood cells and platelets to be low, and neither disappointed. I get the Nesta shot tomorrow, and in two or three days, those white cells should rebound. Until then, same old routine—stay indoors, avoid raw fruits and veggies, yada, yada, yada. Platelets are at 37 and have certainly been lower in past cycles, but they are nearly half of last week's counts, and I will get blood rechecked again on Thursday; if the trend continues, I may need an infusion of turkey gravy, or platelets. My red blood cells are still in good shape—11.7 and 35.6 for hemoglobin and hematocrit, respectively. Relatively speaking, the roller-coaster ride is a little less dramatic this cycle, just a general feeling of the blahs without the dragging bottomless pit of exhaustion. Tired and puffy, but manageable—so far.

I have noticed a new round of faces during the last few visits to my doctor's office, and across all age groups, not necessarily the elderly. And what's more disturbing to me is I haven't seen a few familiar faces for a while; perhaps the two delays in my treatments have thrown my schedule off with others, but I do know at least two of these patients have died. This is the reality of cancer.

I asked one of the nurses if it was difficult for them to see their patients die; I even wondered to myself as I was asking this how often they have been asked this very question or how often people think to ask but hold back, afraid to trespass onto their painful or personal turf. The nurse replied calmly, reflectively, that sometimes it can be difficult, but considering the pain endured by some patients who have challenging conditions or cancers with low survivability, it is a relief to see them pass on and be at peace, for their sake and the sake of their families. And, of course, the many more success stories help impact the losses; it's a balance, she said. She paused, looked down for a moment, and in that silence, I saw sadness, but acceptance. Her eyes then reached up to mine, and she smiled reassuringly (for me or for her, I am not sure). "Of course, that is why we love to see you doing so well." She got up and left the room and my heart and soul followed her, leaped onto on her back and gave her a big, warm hug that I hope she felt the rest of the day.

The circle of life is a continuum, a guarantee from Mother Nature, a promise from God (no matter the form in which one celebrates or what one calls this Higher Power). As I pondered the vast variability and unpredictability that illness and cancer presents in that life continuum, I received an e-mail this afternoon announcing that a friend had given birth to a beautiful, healthy baby girl this past weekend. Attached to the e-mail was a picture of this brown-eyed bundle of joy, a reminder of the life-continuum promise of renewal, hope, and all good things possible. I see the incredible happiness (and relief) this friend feels as she holds her precious child, and my heart melts at the pureness, the sacredness and celebration of new life. And there is so much more in that picture than a proud new mom, because I know my friend's story, and that in this picture she is also a daughter who is thinking about her own father, who is battling cancer. I think to myself how poignant this moment in life must be for her and her dad. The drumming, rhythmic heartbeat of the ebb and flow of life is ever present and accessible to us at any time when we stop in silence to listen. I find comfort and reassurance in the silence, feeling the drumbeat of our eternal souls. Here, there is no separation in being human, and our connection to one another is undeniable. I cannot tell you how much that brings me joy.

As I transition my journey from the battle to the cured, from the days, weeks, and months of focus on the physical healing to stepping— *leaping*—over the line to active, planned participation in work, a healthy lifestyle, and new goals (writing, volunteering, *actually living*), I hope I do not lose this accessibility, this feeling, this direct line to the eternal, natural connectedness of life. I find comfort and peace here, and of course, the great leveler—humility. I hope I do not get so caught up (again) in the distractions of the material world and everyday trivialities that I forget the way to this path. For me, the spiritual security net of human connectedness is where truth, pure creativity, and potential exist and spring forth. For lack of a better word (as if "lack" has anything to do with it), it is—*love*. And from here, all things are possible.

Another Complication

I knew when I awoke this morning that something wasn't right. I went to bed last night starting to feel the body crash, accompanied by sore, achy, knotty muscles. I received the growth shot yesterday, and my right arm was bruised from the shot; pain emanated up the back of my arm into my back and neck. I took Vicodin last night to dull the pain so I could finally sleep. This morning, I was more lethargic than I had felt in a very long time, and I really had to push myself to get ready to go to the doctor's office for a blood draw. Although my red blood cells are still in decent shape, my white blood cells are even lower at .07. (Translation: I have only 70 white blood cells per cubic millimeter of blood; a normal count is between 4,100 and 10,000.) And my platelets have dropped to 7. I have been here before, with even lower red blood cells, and yet I have not felt this lethargic. I also had a fever of 100.9. I could barely keep my eyes open, my energy level was so low.

Neutropenic is the term used for *dangerously* low white blood cells. I have managed through this condition each cycle without needing antibiotics—until now. A patient in this condition who also feels run-down may be suffering from an infection that the body cannot fight without the necessary amount of white blood cells, and the next step is usually a hospital admittance, which involves receiving antibiotics and lots of fluid via IV. There is also a concern about exposing someone in this condition to the airborne illnesses and viruses that abound in a hospital setting. Because of that, my doctor is trying to manage my condition through his office, allowing me to stay at home and thereby reducing my exposure to these illnesses. Ironically, members of his staff are getting over a cold that has been plaguing them for the last couple of weeks, and many patients in his office are also ill (as far as I can tell from the many coughs I hear from the treatment area). One of the nurses told me there is an epidemic of "C-Diff," a strain of virulent diarrhea that is highly contagious and very hard on the body, going around the hospital.

I was hooked up to an IV in the doctor's office to receive my first dose of antibiotics. Chris then pushed me in a wheelchair (I was too weak to walk) over to the infusion center to receive platelets. Next, I was back at the doctor's office to receive potassium and saline to hydrate my body. The nurse swabbed my throat to test for strep and drew more blood to test for staph infection. It takes twenty-four to seventy-two hours for results; if they're positive, I'll be treated with an antibiotic specific to that strain. I was told to return to the doctor's office on Friday for more antibiotics and fluid, and then report to the infusion center on Saturday and Sunday for the same treatment. All of this is due to the very harsh impact of chemotherapy on the body, putting my immune system in a compromised state and making me susceptible to infection. It seems very cruel and unfair, this late in my treatments, with an upcoming PET scan which could declare me cancer-free, that I should be teetering on the edge of a serious infection or septic shock. But I will face this challenge like I've faced all these diversions, determined to get back on my feet and beat this thing once and for all.

The Cumulative Effect of Chemo
November 2008

Expect the unexpected. You would think I would have learned this by now. These later cycles, at least going several days into them, are getting tougher. Even though my overall red blood cell counts have stayed in a higher range (which tells me I am winning this fight), the chemo assault on all my good cells is taking its toll. The cumulative effect of the drugs in my system is wreaking havoc on me physically and emotionally. What has changed, I believe, is that most (if not all?) of those darn cancer cells are gone, so the chemo has nothing left to attack but all the good ones, and now into my sixth cycle, my body's restorative ability is being severely challenged. The deeper we go into these cycles, the harder it is for my body to maintain its delicate balancing act. Until now, a shot of Nesta was all it took for my body to rebound from having low or nonexistent white blood cells. Now I need assistance. I don't like being pumped up with antibiotics, wiping out every little bug in my system, but I have no choice. My medical team's concern about an infection is real, and although I appreciate the precautions they are taking, I just don't think I have or will catch an infection. For some reason, my mind doesn't want to embrace the seriousness of that, but I am following all the medical steps necessary—although not without some feeling of inconvenience. My doctor told me I should expect to receive antibiotics and other necessary fluids intravenously through Tuesday, maybe beyond.

I now know what they mean when weeks, months ago they told me this particular chemotherapy treatment is very aggressive. Y'all ain't kidding. I have only occasionally thought about how I will need to physically restore my body when all of my treatments are done, but thinking about it is no longer a luxury; I must set about creating a very serious plan, because I cringe to think what the chemo drugs and antibiotics are doing to me in the long run. Of course, this by no means diminishes the fact that these very drugs are saving my life.

I need to find humor out of the mental morass of the depression I find myself feeling at this stage because my body is so unrecognizable to me. Self-deprecating humor is a tool I use, although too much of it can get me even more depressed. It is a horrific sight, my naked body. I sometimes cannot help but stare at myself in disbelief and amazement. Think "white aborigine pigmy." To get a laugh out of my husband, I'll sometimes flex my muscles and do that signature Incredible Hulk anger pose to accentuate my puffed-up arms and shoulders and neck. Chris put his hand on the hump at the top of my back, right at the base of my neck, and asked me what that was. It's all water and fat retention, so much of it, around mostly my midsection, face, neck, and back, that some of it just doesn't know where to go. Thus, I've got this charming hunchback effect going on. I told him I look like a turtle. Other than this metamorphosis, there is a physical feeling of bloatedness and just plain yuckiness. This morning, I told Chris that I feel like I'm wearing a full-body blood pressure cuff that's wrapped around me from head to toe, pumped up with air, and squeezing me all over. If I could just have someone peel back the Velcro from the cuff, all the air would escape and the normal me would step out.

Self-deprecating humor aside, I do look in the mirror and see my brown eyes, my spirited soul staring back at me with recognition. And my husband sees this, too. His reassuring hugs, kisses on my bald head, and the fact that he will still hold me for hours on end while we're sitting on the couch makes all of this endurable. I cannot let that kind of love down. I have a responsibility not just to myself, but to this man who loves me without condition, to restore my healthy self—in mind, body, and soul. He deserves no less than that.

The Me Yet to Come

I sing the Body Electric
I celebrate the me yet to come
I toast to my own reunion
When I become one with the Sun

I was humming that tune in my head this afternoon. It's a song from the musical *Fame*. It just popped into my head, in a timely fashion, of course. I had my PET scan today, and I feel I am marching closer toward that path of recovery and renewal. The words of that refrain from the song "I Sing the Body Electric" are very appropriate. *Fame* is one of those uplifting musical films that my siblings and I would watch over and over as we were growing up, singing along with the songs. I haven't seen the movie in probably more than twenty years, but I can still remember just about every song from it.

Today was a long day, involving the PET scan and more antibiotics and fluid. My sister was with me all day; Chris is traveling through Thursday. The nurse told me that I indeed have an infection, although she didn't know the specifics. That information is left to the doctor to review with me, and apparently he didn't have time to see me today, but will tomorrow. They will continue to give me antibiotics each day through Friday, which should knock out the infection. My counts are also higher, and overall I am feeling better than last week, but still tired and worn out. Yesterday, the nurse had told me that this could be my last cycle. She says that, with the issues I've had the last couple of cycles, my bone marrow may be letting us know that it is reaching its limit for the chemo's intensity. If I do have more cycles, she said it may be just one or two more, and the doctor might give more time in between or reduce the dosages. But from their estimations, the end of the treatments is near. Of course I am very excited, but not overly so—my energy level is still so low and, frankly, I don't want to set my expectations too high. I am also quite confident of my absolute recovery, so regardless of what the PET results show, I know I will do the necessary steps to be free from this disease.

It's Election Day. I thought the timing of my PET scan on this day was uncanny. And I'm also glad I voted early, since my days are unpredictable. Today would not have been a good day for me to be standing in a long line, as if I would have had the time anyway. But change and renewal abound on this day, and there is plenty of hope to go around. Again, that song above circulates in my head; and this time I sing it not from my own vantage point, but from a "we," "our" perspective, and it has a greater meaning. Hope springs eternal, no matter the outcome.

Courting Freedom

Cancer-free? Although not official, it's looking real good. Today, I received results of the PET scan, even though the doctor was not completely prepared for our discussion, having received the written report just minutes before our meeting. What he told me is that there has been significant reduction in the diseased lymph node sites, indicating they are clear of cancer. What is inconclusive, he said, is the bone marrow result. Because I received a growth shot last week, which stimulates white blood cell production, that bone marrow activity showed up on the PET scan, essentially masking the ability to see the progress in the diseased area. According to my doctor, he thinks I'm in good shape and done with any further treatments, but he didn't want to get my hopes up completely without fully analyzing all the data. He will review the notes and the actual scans this weekend and wants me to come back next week to discuss his conclusions. He also said he will have me schedule another bone marrow biopsy, the results of which will help him determine if I am cancer-free and no longer need further chemotherapy. *Fantastic news!*

Because of the infection that they have been treating, I was already given next week as an extra week off before starting the next round of chemo, if it was necessary. This will give me time to see him for this follow-up and to schedule the bone marrow biopsy. I asked him how long the drugs will stay in my system once I am done with chemotherapy. He said it will take weeks for my body to process the drugs, for the puffiness to go away, and for my stamina to be regained. In the meantime, he said, go out and celebrate this weekend. Woo hoo!

Chris, Michael, and I left the doctor's office to go to lunch. It wasn't until I was sitting in the car that the news hit me, and tears started flowing. Of course I expected to have made significant progress, but the reality of this incredibly challenging phase actually coming to a conclusion overwhelmed my senses. Very soon, I will have no more days of total exhaustion, no more days of being in a mental haze of fuzziness and depression, no more days of gastritis, no more days of tight, knotted muscles, no more days of mouth sores or nosebleeds, no more days of constipation and hemorrhoids, no more days of puffiness and water retention, no more days of fearing infection, no more days of a tight chest and rapid heart rate and high blood pressure, no more days of blurry vision, and no more days of blood-pressure-cuff body suits. I have been tested, and I'm *this close* to getting a passing grade. I am almost at a loss for words—me, of all people—to fully express the significance of this news, but I see the light at the end of the tunnel, and it is getting brighter and brighter, rushing in the dawn of a new me. Look out, world, here I come!

Illuminating Souls

Chris has a new pet name for me: Uncle Fester. Fabulous. Remember Uncle Fester from *The Addams Family*—the bald, fat uncle with dark circles under his eyes? Chris says all I need is a light bulb to put in my mouth, and I'm sure the chemo residue would light it up just fine. Humor—you must have plenty of it. I guess I can take it coming from my husband, since he's the one who has to kiss Uncle Fester good night and wake up to him in the morning; so far, he's not complaining.

I had a rather busy social weekend. Saturday night, we had plans to go to the opera with our friends Alex and Alex (married couple with the same name). I wasn't sure any of my dressy outfits would fit me, so I decided to go to the mall, and going to the opera is a perfect reason for a new outfit anyway. I did my best to contribute to the economy that day, and I wondered to myself what economic recession were we in with all the parking lots full and the mall packed with shoppers. I really didn't see many people at the cash registers, however. Maybe folks just needed to get out and about; it's been such a dreary few weeks and months for the nation. And with gas prices cut in half from this past summer, hopefully that will translate to some financial relief for many people and businesses to help spur on an economic recovery. We shall see, but I did my part.

At home, I put on my new dress, shoes, and coat, and Chris and I were off to dinner and the opera with the Alexes. We had never been to the opera before; this was a virgin experience for all of us. It was *Madame Butterfly*, and we were quite relieved to have an electronic translation available to us at our seats so we could follow along with the Italian lyrics. My overall impression is that opera must be like wine: one must acquire a taste for it. I am still in the acquiring stage. Speaking of wine, I had my first full glass of an awesome red Bordeaux at dinner. Alcohol had been off-limits during treatment, except for an occasional sip of wine I would steal from my husband's glass the past several months. We dined at a French restaurant, and I ordered steak. The red wine was a particularly great match. I could have jumped into my glass and bathed in the velvety richness of the peppery, smoky berry nectar. It was that good. I have clearly acquired a taste for wine, so maybe the opera isn't too far behind.

Sunday, I met a few girlfriends for brunch. We set this date up weeks ago, and I so appreciate that they tried to schedule a day that would coincide with the good days in my cycle. (That's also why we picked this weekend to attend the opera.) We had a great time catching up—so much so that a couple hours at brunch wasn't enough, and with some more good storytelling still left, but no alcohol served at the restaurant, we decided to walk over to the local pub for an afternoon libation. (Are you starting to see a theme here?) My drink of choice was a Bloody Mary, perfect for a Sunday afternoon of storytelling at a pub, with football on the TV in the background.

I then rushed home to greet an old friend, who also happens to be one of the best bosses I have ever had in my working career. He was in town on business and asked to visit with me and Chris while he was here. We talked for a couple of hours about work, life, and family, and he asked me if there was anything he could do to help me with my recovery, my future. At one point, he asked how my relationship with God has changed through this journey. The three of us had a brief discussion on God and religion in our lives.

Later, I pondered this question. It's interesting how the topic of God and religion continues to come up occasionally with friends, but mostly with family (especially my extended family) and sometimes their fellow church members (strangers to me, but sincere and loving well-wishers in my recovery). I wonder if people are truly curious about my views or are concerned about my soul being saved. I have great respect and admiration for the incredible commitment to faith and God that some of my friends and family have. Their convictions and beliefs and love for God and Jesus clearly center them in their Christian faith. Sometimes I wonder if some of the great blessings and messages I receive from these good Christians have an underlying concern: that I may be lost because I do not belong to a church or profess a particular Christian faith. I would like anyone who feels that way to please rest assured on this: I am not lost. I am on a journey of self-discovery, and a part of that journey is reconnecting and celebrating my personal relationship with God. I consider myself lucky and blessed to have experienced a variety of religious and spiritual teachings throughout my life. I was raised Catholic. That set a foundation for me, yet I hungered for more information and knowledge of other faiths. Over the years, I have had many friends and made acquaintances with people belonging to different faiths (a variety of Christian faiths, and Buddhism, Hinduism, Judaism, Mormon, even atheism), and I learned about each of their unique beliefs and traditions. I found there were similar threads and tenets practiced and taught by these various religions, the most common being love. I have also read many books on religion and spirituality. I continue to be a student on the topic of God, who I believe to be synonymous with truth and love. And I believe God, truth, love, resides within all of us, a singular beam of light straight through our hearts, illuminating our souls, connecting us all to each other. When I envision that light and feel its strength, I am at peace, and I know I am loved and will not be harmed.

There is no doubt in my mind that the many prayers made on my behalf were received and acknowledged. I have felt the energy flowing through me, riding that wave of bright light containing within it all the truth, love, and joy that the universe wishes upon us all and that God bestows on all his children. Only one more hurdle to pass this week (the bone marrow biopsy), and I am free from the struggle. Free to explore and deepen my personal relationships (with God, with friends, with family), free to answer the call for my life's purpose, and free to spread goodness everywhere. Do not worry and pray for my soul to be saved. I am Love. And so are you.

Freedom Crushed

"I've looked over the information and I'm putting in orders for you to have two more cycles," my doctor said as I sat down on the exam table.

"Wh-what? Wh-why?" I was in disbelief, the wind totally knocked out of my sails.

That's how my doctor visit started today. Not at all what I expected after our last discussion when he was leaning toward giving me an all-clear. Over the weekend, he thoroughly reviewed the notes and my chart, along with the PET scan results and did not feel the information was sufficient to stop treatments. He explained to me that not all the lymph nodes are back to normal size; most of them are, but a couple of them, while reduced in size, are still slightly enlarged. Given this, plus the fact that the bone marrow portion is still inconclusive, he does not feel he has enough information to declare me cancer-free. Eight cycles is protocol, he said, and I will need to complete two more cycles. Additionally, he will increase the dosage of one of my chemo drugs. I asked him why, particularly given the fact that my blood counts have been so compromised throughout the treatment. He said he would have ordered this step earlier, but with the issues I was having such as internal hemorrhaging, infection, and my low counts, he had held off. He said, "We need to bite the bullet" (poor choice of words, by the way) and increase the dosage now to give my treatment its best chance of success. I told him my body is really taking a beating, and he acknowledged that I will need to be monitored closely. Great.

At this point, my mind just went to mush. I could have asked more questions, but I was completely deflated. I'm terrified about the prospect of an increased chemo dosage, as I am now living with the cumulative effects of the chemo drugs, and it is, in a word, shitty. I wish I had received this information last Friday. On Friday, I was more prepared for this type of realism. Today, I was ready to leap toward life after chemo and turn the page on this disease. Instead, I was thrown a hand grenade, and my world has come to a loud, ear-splitting, grinding halt. Last Friday, when I was prepared for realism, it took several minutes for the great news of potentially being done with treatments to sink in before I was overwhelmed with joy and started to cry. Today, when I was ready to touch the sky, this unwelcome news punched me square between the eyes, and the tears were immediate. And I've been crying off and on all afternoon.

Chris was with me today, offering words of encouragement, holding me close and drying my tears. He left later this afternoon for a quick overnight trip, and I know he hated leaving me with this disappointing news and my misty eyes and red, dripping nose. I am alone tonight for the first time. We had agreed days ago that this would be okay, since we had thought I was so close to kicking this thing to the curb, but we also thought I'd have better news to keep me company. *C'est la vie.* I will get through this. It is just another climb up the hill on that roller-coaster ride that I've been on since June, with only a few more weeks of unpredictable days of fatigue and feeling lousy. Hundreds of thousands, millions even, have been here before and taken that ride and come out on top. I am just one of many, ready to take my seat next to them and ride into the sunset toward a promising horizon and a healthy new life.

The Weight of Dread

I was down for the count yesterday. A day earlier, I went to get a flu shot and a pneumonia shot, as instructed by my doctor. One shot per arm, upper shoulder. By that evening, I was starting to get feverish, and my right arm where I took the pneumonia shot was getting very stiff and sore. I popped a couple of Tylenol and Vicodin for the pain and went to bed. Yesterday, I awoke with a 101.5 temperature. I called my doctor's office, and he said I was having a reaction to the flu shot; he said to take Tylenol and if I didn't feel better later in the day to call. My temperature fluctuated between 101.4 and 103, and I wasn't feeling any better several hours later, so I called again. My temperature had never climbed this high before, so it alarmed me. He wasn't concerned and was positive I was having a "typical" reaction to the flu shot. I was basically in bed all day long sleeping off and on, just worn out by the fever.

I felt a little better this morning and peeled off my bedding and sheets to wash—I didn't want to sleep in sweaty sheets another night. I was still pretty groggy and didn't have much of an appetite. Finally this afternoon, my temperature dropped to normal levels, and I weaned myself off the Tylenol. But, I just checked it again because I was starting to get the chills, and it's now up to 101.6. I don't get it. More Tylenol—we'll see how that does. My right arm is feeling a little better, but still very sore and stiff. Here I was given an extra week off between cycles, and I'm robbed of a couple of days. I hate that.

Since the roller-coaster news of the last week, I've received a ton of encouraging messages from friends and family telling me to hang in there and be strong. These words are so welcome and healing and helpful to me. Some of the e-mails made me cry, they were so full of wonderful, kind words of support. Yesterday was also the day that phone calls were plenty—I must have received a dozen calls from people checking in on me. Unfortunately, I only had enough energy to get to a couple of them; I was just so out of it.

I'm looking forward to tomorrow night: My family is coming over and we are celebrating Chris's birthday, a few days early. I haven't seen my family in a couple of weeks. Two weeks ago I was too sick, and last week was our opera outing. I look forward to seeing everyone tomorrow night and toasting Chris. We've been singing karaoke the past few gatherings with my sister's karaoke system, a birthday gift from her husband. My family enjoys partaking, but I'm not sure Chris is much of a fan. Of all the things that make him so perfect, carrying a tune is not one of them.

So this weekend is my last weekend of freedom before the chemo assault begins. I have an MRI scheduled Monday afternoon for my upper legs and lower spine. My doctor ordered this test to get a new "baseline" for these areas. Then, Tuesday, we start the routine all over again with cycle seven. They are upping my dosage for one of the chemo drugs that I take on days one, two, and three. I am not sure why the doctor is doing that, since I thought my treatment was already at a maximum for my body weight and height (although I have put on extra weight, hmmm). I really look ahead to this week with much trepidation and dread. This is the first time I have felt this way. I have told many that I would rather be safe and catch every little bad cell, but my tune changed a little with the last cycle, as the chemo drugs are really taking their toll on me. And the mental depression has been building. Perhaps it is time I have a discussion with my doctor about this and maybe get some happy-mental drug help the last few weeks. I have this weekend to enjoy and clear my head. Six more weeks—as long as there are no issues. I can do this. I've made significant progress. Be still and know that I am.

Stealing Moments of Normal

I had an MRI today of my upper legs and lower spine. I was at the imaging center for three hours and in the cave (scanner) for most of that time, listening to the sounds of the honks, horns, and machine gun. The earplugs they provide only partially take some of the edge off the intrusive, unrelenting noises. MRIs are not the most comfortable of procedures, as anyone who has gone through one can attest. You must lie absolutely still for an eternity, and if you are claustrophobic, forget about it. Through the loud noises, I must have been able to doze off occasionally, as the time seemed to go by quickly. Tomorrow, on my husband's birthday, I start cycle seven.

The weekend was fun and relaxing. Saturday night was filled with family visiting and laughter. My sister made chili, and we had carrot cake from The Cheesecake Factory (courtesy of Chris's mom—thank you!). We toasted Chris for his upcoming birthday. My nephew, Kenny, plucked away on his guitar and sang songs to us. A family friend was over, and he also entertained us with his soulful voice. And of course, there was karaoke. It was the best I have felt in a few weeks, the effects of the chemo drugs minimized, and the infection episode and high-fever days behind me (although my right arm was still smarting from the pneumonia shot three days earlier). Sunday was even better, as Chris and I slept in and enjoyed the day together and took a walk in the warm fall sun. I hadn't walked in weeks, and it felt great.

I am so thankful to have these days, surrounded by love and family, celebrating and supporting each other. These moments help me forget my plight, and for a few precious hours, I feel normal. My oldest niece was here Saturday night with her baby, my grand-niece, and as they were leaving, I hugged the twenty-month-old baby and felt her exposed legs and said she needed a blanket. She knew the word *blanket* and immediately nodded yes, instructing me with her big, round, brown eyes to find her one. I grabbed a throw-blanket and wrapped her whole body in it. Her face glowed in appreciation for the security of that blanket, and she gave me a sweet, gentle kiss. And that's what the love of family is like, a giant blanket that wraps you in warmth and comfort, protecting you from the cold, dark night, and helping you feel normal.

CYCLE SEVEN

Tipping Point

A Change in the Air

Days one and two of cycle seven are in the books and behind me. And so far, so good, as my body usually does okay the first week of each cycle. The chemo drug Etoposide (or VP-16), infused on days one through three, was doubled in dosage as promised by my doctor, and the nurse told me to expect an increased chance of nausea. She recommended I use the anti-nausea suppositories that I was prescribed early on in my treatments, and she suggested I insert one at night before I go to sleep.

When chemotherapy started four months ago, I was given three drugs to treat nausea at home. The first two were in pill form. Take pill number one at the first wave of nausea. If pill number one did the trick, then I could continue to take it every four to six hours as needed. However, if the queasiness did not go away after fifteen minutes, then pill number two was the second level of defense. And this one, I could only take every eight hours. After twenty minutes or so of continued nausea, then the third line of defense was the suppository. This, I could only use every twelve hours. Each step up in the level of protection also significantly increased drowsiness. Thankfully, I've mostly relied on the first-level anti-nausea pill, usually on about day four of treatments, and only occasionally have I had to pop a pill of level-two protection.

On the nurse's recommendation, I went straight to the third line of defense and used the suppository last night. It really knocked me out; it's got all kinds of good drugs in it that make you sleepy. She also suggested I take one before coming in for today's treatment, but I decided not to since it made me so groggy. After day two of treatments, I've not experienced any feelings of nausea so far. My good friend Alex joined me today as my "chemo-sabe." (I love this term; I wish I could take credit for it, but I first discovered the word a couple of weeks ago on the blog of a friend's sister who beat cancer earlier this year.)

My doctor was out again yesterday when the results from Monday's MRI came in, and the nurse practitioner gave me a copy of the report. He deferred any analysis to my doctor, but he did say he felt the overall information was positive. What I can glean from the data is that it appears that the bone marrow in my left femur is clear. The diseased area in the right femur is significantly decreased, with an area about 4.5 centimeters that indicates disease. I am not sure how that compares to the earlier scans, and will need to get that information from my doctor.

Another gorgeous fall day today, not a cloud in the sky and nearly seventy degrees in November! We have had splendidly sunny and warm weather like this the past several weeks, give or take a day or two of cold. There is nothing like driving from the east side of metropolitan Denver to the west on such picturesque mornings like today, the sun shining behind you, the crisp, deep-blue skies ahead of you, and the majestic mountains rising up against this beautiful azure canvas. The day is so clear, you can see the shadowy details of the foothills against the mountain range fifteen miles in front of you, the rolling grassy hills, and just beyond that, green pine trees seem to climb the mountain faces, stopping short at about thirteen thousand feet, where the wildflower fields and tundra give way to the rocky tops dusted with snow. It is a sight to behold and another reminder of God's grace.

One more day to revel in this glory before cold, stormy sleet and snowy weather settles in, according to the forecast. But even those gloomy days should be welcomed. They exist to bring in much-needed moisture and help us appreciate breathtaking, warm days like today. Such is the beauty and mystery of Mother Nature and the universe.

Fly, Butterfly, Fly

I made a very difficult decision today. My treatments are extending beyond the short-term disability offered by my current employer, and I have decided to go on long-term disability, which, according to company policy, terminates my employment. I considered taking an unpaid leave of absence so that I could continue to be covered under the company health insurance plan, but with a chronically strained economy and the probability of more layoffs, I didn't think an unpaid status was any safer than a paid one. And frankly, Chris was not a fan of my eventual return, as we both felt the work climate there had turned toxic over the past couple of years. (Five people I know, including me, had cancer, and others suffered from stress-related ailments including insomnia, depression, and high blood pressure.) Therefore, I opted to take advantage of long-term disability, which allows me a percentage of pay until my doctor and I agree on a return-to-work status. The difficulty of the decision is in ending a ten-year run, the longest I have enjoyed at any one company. I built a successful career there, enjoyed solid business relationships, and formed many friendships; my skill set improved, and I was promoted and rewarded well. I did not realize how sad this would make me feel.

So what's on the other side of this decision? Wellness and health and cancer-free, the obvious answer. But I must also embark on the new passion I have discovered for writing and exploring and becoming active in areas that interest me and for which I feel I can make a lasting impact. There is some riskiness in this, unknown income potential, unknown success. But I feel I have been given this opportunity since being diagnosed with this disease. It has just taken me some time to listen and believe enough in myself to take the chance life is giving me.

Yesterday, my brother Michael was my "chemo-sabe" for the day, and as I discussed the job situation before me, he could see the struggle I was still going through arriving at a decision. He understood what bothered me, or rather, what I may have been "fearing"; not so much in leaving a long-term, comfortable situation, but maybe at releasing myself to be truly great at something else. He told me about a scene from the movie *Coach Carter*, and promptly he surfed the Net for the particular quote he was looking for. In the movie, Coach Carter challenged his students about what they feared, and one of the main characters in the movie stood up and answered with the following poignant soliloquy:

> Our deepest fear is not that we are inadequate. Our deepest fear is that we are powerful beyond measure. It is our light, not our darkness that most frightens us. Your playing small does not serve the world. There is nothing enlightened about shrinking so that other people won't feel insecure around you. We are all meant to shine as children do. It's not just in some of us; it is in everyone. And as we let our own lights shine, we unconsciously give other people permission to do the same. As we are liberated from our own fear, our presence automatically liberates others.

I never saw the movie, but this passage was powerful, and Michael knew exactly what I was feeling. I am on my way to finding greatness, which exists in all of us. It serves no one if I hide in the shadow of this realization and retreat from what would make my heart truly sing. It is difficult taking that leap, as my practical and pragmatic side seeks security and protection and wants to find ways to hold on to that which is familiar. But it is time to let these wings soar, to take a chance and follow my dreams and passions, to face the light with a smile on my face, a knowing in my heart, and trust that all will be well.

Giving Thanks

Whew. Okay. Time to rest. I've been taking it easy most of the weekend, tending to domestic chores around the house. With the extra chemo dosages last week, I'm trying to maintain a positive mental attitude in order to keep ahead of the anticipated increased fatigue from this supercharged assault on my blood cells and marrow. So far, I think I am winning the battle, keeping the extra fatigue and worsening symptoms at bay. Of course, as soon as I broach this topic, the roller coaster will sweep me up. Expect it. My hope is that I can time a transfusion on Wednesday, if it is needed, so I can enjoy Thanksgiving with my family. Maybe I'll be surprised to find none is needed. That's probably a little more than I can ask for.

We also have our good friends Jackie and Steve visiting, and they'll be staying with us for a few days beginning on Wednesday. So, I have extra incentive to psych myself into a great mental and physical state of being. Hopefully, Chris will be done with the impromptu home improvement project that has been calling his name for the past couple of weeks: tiling our master bathroom floor. When we purchased our home, the bathroom floor was carpeted, and nearly five years later, we are finally doing something about it. Of course, we had no choice after we discovered a few weeks ago that mold and other lovely bugs decided to move in under the carpet around the shower. Certainly not welcome visitors, and definitely not for someone with an already depressed immune system.

As Thanksgiving approaches, there is so much to be thankful for this year. I find my mind is fixated on these blessings and tossing each one of them around in my chemo-hazed brain, as I try to focus on giving them their due, while thinking ahead to the future when I can claim victory over this illness and begin a challenging new career. There is much that is not known—an understatement, to be sure. And that is where faith takes over. I long for the days of clear-mindedness, when I can piece together not just one or two hours of productive mental activity, but a day's worth. I miss my active mind. I miss my active body. But the pace of healing is necessary and cocoons me from complete insanity and wasting away. Life is always happening, so boredom has rarely been my partner through this, and I am taking things one step at a time. After all, it takes everything you've got to focus on recovery, and aside from moments of frustration from this slowed-down pace, I am grateful it is what I can manage. I am thankful to be alive.

My Knight in Shining Armor

Knock. Knock.
Who's there?
"Mini-Me."
"Mini-Me" who?
"Mini-Me" who shows up when you can't quite fill out the shell of your body.

Fatigue has settled in my body tonight, but I am not deterred. It is just low blood counts. I don't feel the grip of anything like the staph infection from the last cycle that left me feeling very lethargic and had me receiving intravenous antibiotics for eight straight days in the doctor's office; nor do I feel the onset of flu symptoms or a fever—all good signs. I am pleasantly surprised that I have not crashed too hard with the extra chemo dosage from last week, although I do realize I have just completed day eight today, and the effects of the chemo are still working on my body as I write this. All of my counts are compromised, white blood cells the most—again. Platelets are depleted but hanging in there, and I will need that checked again in a few days. The red blood cell counts dipped as I anticipated they would, and I'll need a couple of units tomorrow. That transfused mojo should pep me right up, just in time to enjoy Turkey Day with the family.

Yes, this fatigue has me feeling like I am strung out on drugs and, as long as I don't push it and get plenty of rest, my senses won't overload and I won't "go postal," like I did today on my poor husband as we were leaving the doctor's office. Right there in front of the elevator, in public. Chris, as many know, is truly a saint. He works hard, and when he can, he accompanies me to my appointments, laptop and Blackberry in hand, still working and making phone calls. When he is in that zone, I am—well, invisible. When he is out of that zone, he then decides to take charge of me. Which he did, in front of the elevator as we were leaving the doctor's office. When he takes charge of me, his nonverbal communication skills just take over and I somehow need to recognize that that is when I am supposed to give over all control to my wonderful husband. So that when I ask a question, it is moot, you see, because he is in charge and doesn't need to answer it. It is irrelevant. He is in charge. Very damsel-in-distress on the one hand, ya know, like in the silent movies, the man in charge coming to the rescue of the lady tied down on the railroad tracks. And very irritating on the other hand. At least in the silent movies there are cue cards that communicate the action and dialogue. When my husband takes charge, he oftentimes forgets the cue cards. Get me a teleprompter, please. But I know this about him. I love him despite it and can generally navigate the torturous cone of silence when my simple questions go ignored. However, as I slip deeper into fatigue and "Mini-Me" mode, being ignored is way too much for my senses to handle, especially having expended the energy to not only think of the "irrelevant" question on my drug-hazed mind, but to then verbalize it, *and not to mention that I was starving*; and thus, the reasons for my going postal in front of the elevator. And this is the amazing thing about my husband: he takes the verbal assault, quietly, probably thinking to himself, *My poor, cancer-challenged wife is having an emotional outburst*, and remarkably, he is cool and calm. And this is why I love him even more. He takes me, all of me, outbursts and all, and will still lean over and kiss me on the top of my head. So what if he ignores my irrelevant questions? He is in charge, and all is well.

Tonight, Saint Christopher is at it again, working on the damn bathroom floor and challenging my "Mini-Me" status once more. I am on drugs, for goodness' sakes. Nevertheless, I assist as he asks, looking up on the Internet various how-to instructions for this and that. Tonight it is for mixing and laying grout. After much hemming and hawing—Do we have enough grout? How long will this take?—we decided much-needed sleep was in order, particularly since he stayed up until 1:30 this morning completing the mortar portion of the tile project from hell. He will finish off just enough of an area for us to have the room functional so that we can get to bed earlier than the wee hours of the morning, and the home improvement project will then need to take a rest for a few days before absolute perfection and completion. The project seems to be reflecting my current state of being: one step at a time, take a rest when needed, no need to push it, all in due time.

Knock. Knock.

Who's there?

Your husband.

Your husband who?

Your husband who loves you very much—and is "in charge."

Ever Present

Dear Daddy,

It's Thanksgiving today, and you were the topic of much conversation around the dinner table at Jeanette and Ken's house. So many of our favorite memories involve you; you are missed more than you know. But as the stories kept coming and the funny tales poured off the sweet lips of your children and grandchildren, your presence was felt. You continue to live on in our hearts and minds.

So much has happened since you left, eight years, four months, twenty-seven days ago. At least you lived to see the new millennium, and that the year 2000 did not create the predicted computer malfunctions that would halt the world as we knew it. But, thankfully, you did miss 9/11 and the terror attacks that changed the face of this country and the world.

You have a new great-granddaughter, your first, who is twenty months old and carries the same sweetness and goodness of her mother, who twenty-seven years earlier you unselfishly held in your arms and loved without condition as she struggled in her first few days to survive. Remember when we all thought she would die? Of course you do. Angella, your first granddaughter, born to your eldest, Jeanette (herself barely an adult)—and what an "angel" she was to our family. I think Angella's brush with death was the moment our family truly bonded. I mean, we were definitely tight growing up, but that scare defined us as a family, was our first true test with the fragility of life, and we have been braving the world together ever since.

I wonder how you would handle my illness. At times I am glad you are not here to witness this, as I think it would break your heart, seeing your brave little girl face such a health challenge. And so that is why I am convinced you brought me my own angel in my husband, Chris. You worked behind the scenes and fluffy clouds, hand-picked this man, who is so similar to you in kindness and gentleness, to love me and care for me, to carry me through this burden in your place. I often wonder how I could have made this journey without him. You have reached beyond our world to save me. He does not know you, but seeing him sit at the table today and laugh with us as we relived our stories about you, I am sure he has come to know you through our eyes and cherished memories; you could have been sitting there at the table with us—and you probably were.

In fact, as I ponder this possibility even more, it only makes sense that you have never left our side, but have been with us all along: in the cool breeze on a warm summer's day; in the giggles and laughter in your grandchildren's voices; in the calming whisper of the changing seasons; in Mom's silent prayers as she lay flowers at your grave; in my husband's gentle kisses on the top of my head; in the hospital room with me when I learned of my diagnosis. And you were there days later when I was home from the hospital and collapsed in Jeanette's arms, sobbing uncontrollably, reality closing in on me and terrified of the path ahead; you held us both, embraced us with your love. You are there when I get my chemo and blood transfusions, when I can't sleep at night, and when I am too exhausted from the fight. You breathe life into me every moment of the day.

And so on Thanksgiving, it is only appropriate to give thanks to you, for our memories with you and for your spirit's presence. I no longer need to give you an accounting of what's been going on, because you have missed nothing. You have always been here, watching over us, comforting us, loving me, forever holding me in your arms.

Thank you, Daddy, for raising a family with such amazing warmth and love, for showing us the true meaning of life, and for never leaving our side.

Love always,
Barb

Necessary and Beautiful

It's day thirteen of cycle seven, and I'm pretty worn out. Usually, I am on an upswing at this point in my cycles, but I guess the extra chemo and the cumulative effects are gaining an upper hand, despite having two units of red blood cells last Wednesday and two units of platelets on Friday. My white blood cell count was still extremely low on Friday, at .4 (nonexistent, again), but I expected Nesta to kick in at any moment. And after a rough weekend, tonight I am getting more sluggish and my fever is high again. Perhaps I tried to do too much this Thanksgiving holiday, as I took advantage of every burst of energy I could will from my tired shell. Maybe I ate too much rich food, and I probably should have stayed away from the wine! In any event, I'm a little concerned I may have an infection lurking somewhere, and I really don't want to go through eight days of antibiotics via IV again.

Days earlier, the nurse scheduled me to go into the infusion center for a blood draw on Saturday, specifically to check my platelet level, but I could tell on Thanksgiving that my levels were really low, as I was bruising pretty easily and my nose bled from time to time. So, I rescheduled the blood draw for Friday morning, one day early, and good thing I did, because my platelet count was at 11. The practice director (PD) was on call when the infusion nurse called him with the results, and he ordered two units of turkey gravy. (*How timely*, I thought, *the day after Thanksgiving.*) My doc usually orders only one unit of platelets, generally because these cells have a very short life, lasting two to three days in the body, at which point your production should kick in. My doc is more conservative; the PD is a little more aggressive. The PD also instructed me to come in Monday for another blood draw. I am hoping I can tolerate the crappy way I feel just one more night and that it doesn't get worse and send me to the ER.

Geez, is it the end of January 2009 yet? That's my target date for hearing the "all clear," to start feeling like a normal person again, for participating with full gusto and enthusiasm in life. I cannot deny the challenge the treatments continue to be, and how much more difficult it is getting, but I also cannot let it negatively impact my psyche and pull me further down. The tug-of-war is intense.

To focus on the positive, I had one of the most memorable Thanksgiving holiday weekends ever. How can I not be encouraged by my progress, my introspective journey, discovering the incredible bonds of love with family and friends? These wonderful gifts are life-changing and continue to hold me up through these difficult days. It was amazingly fulfilling to sit around the dinner table at my sister's house, with family all around, listening to fantastic stories and memories of my father and of our days growing up together. And for a few hours, the struggles with health were sidelined.

Adding to this most memorable weekend was the visit by our wonderful friends Jackie and Steve from Chattanooga. I have known Jackie for eighteen years, and we have some juicy stories on each other that I am sure we'd prefer to keep to ourselves. She has been married to Steve now for seven years, and she said it best the other night at dinner, "We are all like family." She's right. When you know someone for that long, when you and your husband feel at ease with them, can share all your dreams, goals, desires and know that despite your human imperfections and flaws you are accepted without judgment and loved beyond all measure, then that is synonymous with family. Knowing I am surrounded by these selfless, complete human and spiritual beings helps to make these harsh physical and mental days tolerable and acceptable and necessary—and beautiful.

The Hell of Cancer
December 2008

I am on my cancer-is-a-bitch warpath. The past few days have worn me out, and I just want off this miserable ride. Just a few more weeks of this freaking insanity, I know, but I am so over it! My body is being pushed to the limit. A cold, fevers, raw stomach and bloatedness, mouth and gum tenderness, and overall general malaise and fatigue are stacking the deck against my positive outlook, and I just want to scream. And today I went off prednisone, so with my body crashing, it's adding more intensity to the blazing trail on my warpath.

I was at the doctor's office yesterday and today for a blood draw and hydration. With the pressure in my tummy, I am not drinking the amount of water and fluids I normally do, so I asked for a liter of saline solution both days. My counts today are a mixed bag, with white blood cells finally up at 6.6, but hemoglobin slipped to 10.2 from 11.4 yesterday, and platelets are down to 13 from 22. Those two units of platelets from Friday are all but gone from my system, and my nose is beginning to bleed again. I come back for another blood draw on Thursday, but I have already alerted my doctor of my desire to delay the next cycle another week. I just cannot see myself starting chemo again next week. No way. I want a break.

Chris ended up canceling his business trip, the first time he has done so since starting his new job this past summer. Even he was concerned about me and how run-down I've been feeling and didn't want to leave until he knew I was okay. I am getting through the day with a little help from my friend Vicky (Vicodin), which has me a little happy and groggy, and had me drunk-dialing a few people this afternoon. The Vicodin is taking the edge off the achiness and pain, relaxing me somewhat, but not quite doing the trick for my mental state of mind. With just a few more weeks left in this life-changing journey, I am trying my best to hang on without the aid of antidepressants, although days like these can be a mental obstacle course.

And as always, whenever I reach these low points in my tired struggle, positive messages seem to come my way, either conjured up by my own sheer determination not to be swallowed up by my own misery, or from other outside forces rescuing me from the fiery depths of hell. I was watching *The Ellen DeGeneres Show* and one of the guests was an extraordinary young woman born to this world without any arms. This incredibly brave soul has managed her life without appendages, utilizing her legs and feet in the way we use our arms and hands. As a teenager, she tried prosthetic arms but found them to be more burdensome. She eventually did away with them, preferring her mind-legs-feet connection. She has been quite accomplished in her young life, learning to tap dance and play piano, and as a profession, she is a motivational speaker. Her latest accomplishment is getting a certified pilot's license, the first awarded to a person with no arms. Absolutely amazing. And inspiring.

So I can sit here and wallow in the very real hardship of cancer and the necessary paradoxical chemotherapy treatment, which heals and slaps you down at the same time. And while lately it seems I am having more bad days than good days, all I have to do is remember the real-life heroes in this world who overcome what would be insurmountable for most of us. These reminders prop me up and pull me out of my little pity party. And I am inspired and at peace, as my thoughts transport my body and lay me gently down in a field of wildflowers, flowing up to the base of tall majestic purple mountains and clear cobalt blue skies, where I am wrapped in the warmth of the sun. And for a moment, I forget the hell of cancer and I am healthy, normal, whole.

Hairy Questions

Why is the hair on my legs growing? It's not growing anywhere else. My bald head still holds a few strands on top that sweep over to the left—the ultimate comb-over—which I have not wanted to trim down or shave. I'm hanging on to every last strand on my head that wants to stay. "Screw the chemo," the brittle brown threads say, "we are staying put!" But the hair on my legs, well, those strands I am quite alright shedding, which they did months ago and stayed away for the longest time, but for the last month, they have been sprouting. I have shaved once, and I really don't want to shave again; don't want to encourage them to grow. And if they're growing there, why not on my head? Such are the perplexing questions for the bodily changes that take place while you're on chemotherapy.

Facial hair has been even more perplexing. For more than a couple of months now, I have had to trace eyebrows in place where none exist. It took a while for all the tiny eyebrow hairs to fall out completely, and for weeks, a precious few strands barely linked to form a faint outline of where to draw the brow. Now the chain is gone, only a random wisp here or there, and drawing the brows is a guessing game. Each time I apply makeup, I take the eyebrow pencil and say to myself, "I think that's where this one starts," and the artistry begins. Sometimes I get it right; other times, one brow is obviously higher than the other; sometimes the arch is too severe; and sometimes I use too much pencil and they're too dark and thick. I don't start over. I just sigh. They never look natural, and I feel like Phyllis Diller. And my eyelashes? Those fell out over time, often landing right in my eyes, which was annoying as I rubbed them out. And now that I have none, I get other things in my eyes like dust and other minute particles, things that a full set of lush lashes are supposed to help keep out. Ah, more sighs. Even though waxing is one of those abhorred female necessities, I cannot wait for the day when I find myself on my esthetician's table, on my back, legs spread, eyes blinded by the bright light of the magnifying lamp, ready to feel the torturous pain, a prelude to the perfect bikini line and sexy, arching brow. Because that will mean I have hair again. And that will mean I am healed.

I am feeling better today. I swear these last few days of each cycle, when the chemo is accumulating its nasty effects and the prednisone is building in my body and causing weight gain and discomfort and pressure, are getting harder and harder to navigate. Only one more of these damn cycles to go, only one more of these hellish periods to go through. My head is a little clearer, the tummy and mouth pains have subsided; the head cold and fatigue remain, but that, I can handle.

I went in for a blood draw today, and all counts are good, except platelets continue to be challenged and are only at fourteen—not much changed from Tuesday. So tomorrow I am going for another unit of gravy. And wouldn't you know, my doctor is out again and is gone through all of next week! He was supposed to let me know today if I get to take next week off from chemo. I told the nurse I was going to make the executive decision myself. I'll be back in the office on Monday for another blood draw to check platelets. I am pretty sure I'll get that week off, just like my doctor decided to take!

O Christmas Tree

We decorated our Christmas tree last night with the much-needed help from family. In a little over an hour, we had the baubles and ribbons adorning our faux pre-lit tree—lickety-split, record time! A perfect tree every year, it has been with me and Chris since the first Christmas in our house, four years ago. That year, we hosted the holiday party of all holiday parties, titled it "Bring Your Balls—er, Christmas Ornament," and as the name suggests, we asked that guests bring an ornament to dress our tree. I thought this holiday-themed party would be a great way to amass many ornaments at one time and to help us decorate our barren tree. Friends and family came, each with unique ornaments, some truly gorgeous, others truly garish, and some just hysterical.

Last night, as in past years, each box we opened released memories from that hoppin' holiday party, where we served spiced wine and a decadent spread of food and laughed with friends and family until our faces hurt. We collected more than forty ornaments during that evening four years ago, and for the most part, I can still remember who brought what. This beautiful green-glass ornament was from Rachel; it came in a gold Chinese food box. Alex and Alex brought the red one from Cabo San Lucas. Liz's ornament was in a sleek blue velvet box. Gary and Kelley brought the giant-sized red-striped ornament. Mary and Michael brought the ornament that changes color. Rick's friends' contributions were some of the funniest—Larry, Brian, and Steve gave us a gay-themed disco ball ornament (because no tree is complete without one). Chris and I relive that night every Christmas.

My head is finally starting to come out of the chemo daze, and I am feeling a little more clear-headed than most of last week. I am still fairly tired and weak and haven't done much exercising in quite some time. I have been active only with domestic chores, running errands, and/or meeting friends for lunch. I hope to get this week off from treatments so I can add some more physical rigor to my days and strengthen my stamina before starting the last and final (yay!) cycle.

It's been nearly six months since my diagnosis, and I have to stop now and then to take stock of where I've been and what I continue to endure. And when I am completely honest with myself, it has been a very physically challenging few months. I would say it has been the most difficult thing in my life, but I still think the loss of my father was tougher. There was just nothing like that heartache and the empty feeling and sadness that consumed me for almost a year. But as each of these cycles builds on the last and I continue to feel my body weaken even more, this journey is beginning to rival that painful loss of my father as my biggest, boldest life challenge.

Bang Bang

Yesterday I experienced a medical drive-by shooting. Figuratively speaking, of course. I was at the doctor's office for my scheduled blood draw, and the results were good; white blood cells still stable at 6.3, platelets finally rebounding at 73, while hemoglobin dipped to 9.9. Yet, I was still feeling very tired and run-down, and the nurse who knew I had wanted to take this extra week off handed me a calendar schedule that showed the next chemo cycle starting next Monday. At that moment, the practice director (PD) casually walked by on his way out of the office and asked how I was doing and how my counts looked. The nurse showed him my blood results and told him, "We're delaying the schedule one week because she had a rough week last week and felt pretty worn out." And that's when the bullets started flying.

"I wouldn't delay. Get your chemo done this week—your counts are okay," PD says to me. *Bullet number one.*

"Yes, but I have really felt run-down by the latest round of chemo and feel like my body needs some time off," I protested.

"I highly recommend you don't delay. With Hodgkin's, it's really important that you not go off schedule; that impacts the curability rate," he persisted. *Bullet number two.*

"But I've had all kinds of medical issues during my treatments because of the chemo: infections, internal hemorrhaging. I've had other cycles delayed already." I was pleading.

"I know you have. What we read from studies with Hodgkin's patients is that it's really important to keep aggressive and stay on schedule—it's very important in terms of curability. I highly recommend you not delay." *Bullet number three.*

I was very perplexed and agitated at this point. "But my doctor has increased the VP-16 drug—he's doubled it. It's really having an impact on me."

"He's trying to cure you," he said, curtly. *Bullet number four.*

Self-doubt is creeping in at this point, and I am trying to hold back tears. I know that starting chemo this week is too soon for my body. I pressed on, "We're talking starting either this Wednesday or next Monday—*five days.*"

"I highly recommend you not delay, and I'll write that in your chart." *Bullets five, six, seven, eight, nine, and ten.*

And with that, he turned and walked away, and I was sitting there in disbelief, stunned at what just happened, bleeding from my wounds. Even the nurse seemed stunned, then she said that PD had a point about staying aggressive and also added that she felt my doctor would listen more to how I said my body was feeling. I took the calendar she prepared for me and told her I didn't know what to do now, that I'll keep the schedule where it is but talk to Chris to see what he thinks. I told her if I change it back to this week, as PD's bullet assault recommended, I would call her back that day.

I left the doctor's office and went to the ladies' room. I couldn't hold back the tears anymore, and they just streamed down my face. Was I jeopardizing my curability rate with the decision to hold off chemo for *five days?* Was I screwing myself? I didn't know what to think anymore and never felt so much self-doubt. In that moment, I no longer trusted my ability to listen to my body's needs and trust my own decisions. I was reeling and my head was spinning. I felt like a total loser.

I walked out of the building. The wind was cold and howling ferociously, piercing through my hollow body, causing the tears to sting my face. I made it to my car and sat there for a moment, still crying. I pulled myself together as best I could and called my husband. I was reporting to him my blood counts when he interrupted me and asked why I was sniffling. Damn. He knew right away something was wrong. "Because I was crying," I squealed, barely getting the words out, and the tears flowed again. I explained to him what just happened. He was pissed at first, and then, calmly, he talked me off my emotional ledge. He told me to do what my body was telling me to do; he gave me the support and encouragement that I needed.

None of this would have happened if my doctor would have granted me this request at the time I asked it, instead of delaying the answer until he asked me to come back two days later—at which time, he knew he would be gone, but I didn't. And he failed to delegate granting this request to anyone in his absence, leaving me to listen to my body and make the decision myself. And why shouldn't I? Not to mention that during each of my previous delays in treatment—which were at his direction—he did not inform me that such delays would jeopardize my curability rate. And now that *I* am taking a stand based on how my body is feeling to delay a cycle for just five fucking days, it's only *now* that my curability is impacted? Clearly, my doctor and the PD have differing philosophies, and at times, both have terrible communication skills—not just with each other, but with me as the patient who is caught in the middle. I wondered then, was my doctor reprimanded for each time he delayed my treatment? Geez, I would hope not, as both times my body had just gone through a medical issue serious enough to necessitate extra time before the next cycle started. By the PD's own logic, my curability would have already been impacted because of those delays. Yet, no one said anything to me. And only when *I* ask for *five days* am I made to feel that it is who is screwing with my ability to be cured. Ooooo, let the record show! It will be my fault if I am not cancer-free or if I have a relapse at some point. Bullshit.

Across Oceans and Time

I've been crying a lot lately. Not to worry, though. Last night's tears were tears of joy. I received a package yesterday from my Aunt Kathryn in Pennsylvania. The word *glass* was written on all four sides of the box, and I was very intrigued with what was inside. I opened the box, and on top of the carefully wrapped contents was a card. I pulled the card from its envelope and began reading:

My Dear Sweet Girl!

I was cleaning the hutch last week and as I removed these few dishes, I realized maybe it's time to share. I asked Annette if she wanted them to enjoy for a while—she said, "yes, but you should talk about that with Kathy first because I remember she has first choice over me—although, I do think the dishes should go to our brother Kenneth's family in Denver. Why not discuss it with Kathy?" So I did—

Kathryn and Annette are my aunts, sisters to my father, whom they call Kenneth. Kenneth was his middle name. I've always known my father as James Kenneth, and he introduced himself to people in his adult life as Jim. But Kenneth is what my dad's family called him. Kathy is my cousin, Kathryn's daughter. The note continued:

Well—to my delight, Kathy tells me that when you and Chris visited Kathy and Tom in Austin that you very much admired her teacup collection and at that time you expressed a desire to start your own.

I have written about Kathy's collection earlier in this journal. Her collection is truly exquisite and carries many wonderful stories. I read on:

May I have the pleasure of presenting you with the very first pieces purchased for your collection.

How very cool, I thought. And then:

Your dad brought these dishes ...

My heart stopped, and I took a deep breath and held it. The tears flowed on cue. What was in this box was from my father. I blinked away the tears blurring my eyes so I could continue reading the card:

back from the Philippines and gave them to your grandmother. Annette shared that time with them because she was still at home. She remembers your dad holding the cups to the light to show your grandmother the Lady in the Cup. Our mother treasured these beautiful pieces. Now you can, too. We have carefully washed, dusted, and treasured them over the years, so now they will be in your care where they have always belonged.

Love always, Kathryn

Well, now the tears turned to rivers and my nose was dripping like a faucet. I was trying to catch my breath as I excitedly but gently handled each delicately wrapped item and peeled away their packaging to reveal the beautiful pieces inside. One by one, each collectible presented itself to me like a buried treasure of gold, and my father's and grandmother's spirits were brought to life right there in my kitchen.

Around fifty years old, this set was originally made in Japan and included two teapots (one large, one small), two teacups with matching saucers, and four dessert plates. Each one hand-painted, glazed with an orange-rust-colored background and carefully designed with a brown and multi-colored dragon, I could see the individual artistry of each similar, yet unique piece. On each teapot, the dragon's body circles around the pot, the spout serves as its long neck, and the opening at the spout's end is the head and mouth. The dragon is fierce and gorgeous at the same time. And inside each teacup on the bottom is the delicate outline of a woman's face (the mysterious Lady in the Cup).

I envisioned my father, a young man in his twenties, spotting this set in a shop in the Philippines, admiring it and thinking of his mother and knowing she would enjoy its unique and worldly beauty. Was my own mother with him? Did he know her at the time? I cannot wait to ask her. And here they sit on my kitchen table, having been purchased miles and oceans away, hand-delivered by my father and used for many years by my grandmother, who loved this gift from her son, and admired and treasured by my aunts and cousin. Overwhelming.

And now I have my inaugural pieces to start my own teacup collection with accompanying stories and tales. Only this set will surely hold the most special of places in my heart and carry with it the most poignant of stories. The souls of my father and grandmother will always speak to me from these pieces with messages of love.

Honey, it's time to get a curio cabinet.

Consuming Rage

I let out a loud scream this morning as I was waking. I had one of those nightmarish dreams in which I try to yell, and I could tell in my sleep that my body was not going to let my voice be heard. As soon as I awoke, I still had the feelings from the dream fresh in my mind, and I bellowed a blood-curdling scream. Not high-pitched, but definitely loud, it carried with it pent-up energy filled with frustration and anger. Chris nudged me, thinking I was still sleeping and dreaming. This is usually what he does when he hears me mumbling loudly or screaming in my sleep, which occurs about once a month or so. But this time, I screamed when I *knew* I was awake and no longer dreaming. I had never done that before, but as I came into consciousness and knew I was safe in my bed, I still felt so compelled to let my body's voice be heard. What was I dreaming about? It was a stupid dream where my frustration level kept growing over the littlest of things; my sister, my brother, and my husband were all in it. And while the little things they were doing were annoying me and trying my patience, I knew they weren't at all intentional, but maybe careless and without thought. No, I am not angry at my sister, my brother, or my husband. But what this dream and the subsequent "conscious" yell told me is that anger is occupying my mind and my body.

I don't like feeling angry. It drains energy and is probably the most useless of emotions. And just having this emotion makes me feel guilty. Why, I am not sure. So based on how I feel about this emotion, it is no wonder that I don't deal with it very well, suppressing it deep in my subconscious, where it ticks away like a time bomb. I thought about this incident all day today and the obvious question: why am I so angry? And I didn't have to wait long for answers.

First, there's this illness crap, and my looking at basically losing an entire year and more of my life. Tonight is a special anniversary for me and Chris—on this day five years ago, we shared our first get-together (hook-up, actually), and we have been together ever since. And while I looked upon this night with anticipation and much gratitude, I am angry that the last year has been spent being less than a participant, less than a partner in this relationship. Then there's this overall frustration with my doctor's office, the fact that my doctor has been gone a lot during my treatments, that I don't have very much face time with him, that he doesn't have the warmest of bedside manners, that I feel I have to keep on top of all the details concerning my care and communicate that to the staff when they drip my chemo too fast, or don't have the right paperwork on file, that my doctor called me near-clear and then retracted and put me on two more cycles with higher chemo dosage. Yes, yes, I know, he is trying to cure me and probably—no, certainly—has no clue as to how I feel. What's worse is I don't think it would even matter, so I say nothing, and ultimately, that makes me feel of no consequence. And then there's his partner or boss, I am not sure which, the PD, who wounded me pretty good last week by telling me not to delay my last cycle, making me feel like I was compromising my curability rate. And I feel guilty for being angry at them because they are trying to cure me. My life, and the lives of so many others, is in their hands. How could I be so ungrateful?

I am angry at how the treatments and drugs make me feel and look. I am not myself. True, I hadn't been me even months before my diagnosis. But it is difficult living through this, feeling like I can only do a small fraction of the things I used to enjoy, and hating the way that has changed me, robbed me. And being angry over this makes me feel guilty, too, because this is the price for staying alive and being able to one day soon reclaim my health and have the rest of my life. Then there's all the bleakness going on around the world right now, the economic meltdown, the number of job losses piling up every day, the bailouts and the politics and the corruption. And how we're treating our planet and taking each other for granted. I am watching and reading too much of this, but it all makes me angry. And it's Christmastime, always a favorite time of year, always joyous. And I cannot partake. There will be no Christmas cards, no shopping, no holiday parties, no holiday cheer, no caroling, no outdoor lights, no gift-giving. I am too tired. And that makes me angry. And sad.

All of this I am keeping inside, telling no one and sharing with no one this anger, and pushing it to the back of my mind whenever it gets too overwhelming. And so it is no wonder that I have symbolic dreams of growing levels of anger and frustration, and it is no wonder that I scream out loudly as I wake from this dream, realizing that the anger is real and alive inside of me, and I can no longer ignore it and hold it in. I must confront it and figure out a way to deal with it before it swallows me whole.

CYCLE EIGHT

Clawing Out

The Home Stretch

Yesterday was day one of cycle eight, the last chemotherapy cycle—
yippee! My counts are okay, not as high as I would like them, but good
enough to treat. White blood cells were at 4, hemoglobin is at 10.2, and
platelets continue to be challenged at 52. I asked the nurse why that is
lower than last week's 73, having given myself those five extra days to
rebound. She said the chemo is so harsh on the bone marrow that she
has seen patients struggle with platelets for several weeks or months
after treatments have ended. Great. Because of that low count, the nurse
wanted to wait to get PD's approval before starting treatment. We didn't
get the go-ahead until late morning, which had me leaving later than the
other patients, a total of seven and a half hours in the office.

I had a great visit with my dear friend Kelley, who brought down
a scrumptious meal from Whole Foods, a delicious chicken salad and
baguette, topped off by a raspberry dessert bar, and to drink: Orangina.
She asked me if I had ever had Orangina (pronounced "Oran-geena"),
and I said no. It is a drink from England, she said, their version of soda.
It was quite a tasty citrus bubbly concoction. I kept pronouncing it
"Oran-gina," ya know, like "va-gina," and Kelley kept correcting me—it
was quite comical.

As we were eating our meal, the PD and physician's assistant stopped
by for a visit. I wondered if PD remembered his drive-by ambush of
me from last week. But he was in a jovial mood, and he jokingly said,
"We've checked everyone's lunches and decided that yours is the best
and we want it; and since you're getting chemo, we think we can take
you." I laughed, appreciating his attempt at humor. We discussed my
counts, and he made a reference to our conversation from last week. *So
he did remember,* I thought. He talked about the increase in my dosage,
explained that aggressiveness is real important with Hodgkin's because

most of the time they can cure this disease the first go-around by staying on schedule and aggressively treating. So, he was able to soften the blows from last week with his humor and emphasizing that it's their intention to cure me. He also told me to expect to crash in counts, which I do. I actually wouldn't be surprised if I need platelets by Friday, and probably next Wednesday (Christmas Eve), I'll need a couple of units of mojo. Then our conversation turned back to food, and he commented again about how great our meal looked. I asked him if he had ever had "Orangina." And Kelley interrupted, "Oran-geena." (Yeah, by the look on his face, clearly my version didn't sound so appetizing.)

A Strong Fabric

My friends continue to anchor and support me and provide for some very humorous moments as I take my last steps through treatment and edge my way ever so closer to recovery. It is so near, I can taste it.

Last night was our annual BOTS (Books on the Side) book club holiday party. Six of the nine members gathered as we celebrated our friendships, the season. Earlier today, I received two units of blood (days earlier than I thought I would need them), and those precious cells helped keep me somewhat alert during the evening and enjoy the stories and company of these lovely muses in my life. We "Skyped" two of our BOTS members living in other states, getting the chance to see their gorgeous smiles and catch up through the glory of technology. We squealed with delight when Mindy announced she's pregnant with her third child. She looked fabulous, always does. One of the funniest moments came when Rachel commented that Mindy still has "ITC." "What is ITC?" I asked. "Inner thigh clearance!" Rachel enthusiastically proclaimed. I laughed until my face hurt. I'm not sure I've ever had ITC. And there was a lot of toasting going on: a nod toward my ending treatments with my health reclamation in sight, and grand plans for 2009 that involve all of us seeing each other more. I love these times with my friends.

Earlier in the week, I received from my dear friend Christiane a holiday CD she personally created. (Aside from a fantastic hairstylist and budding cattle herder, she is a Martha Stewart wannabe.) The songs are fantastic, country in style, with some Christmas lounge-style thrown in. With it was a Christmas card, also customized with her usual lighthearted, creative humor.

And accompanying this card was a very sweet, handwritten, personalized note from Christiane, and then this perfect quote, which she printed on a bookmark for me to cherish always:

> *Any woman who sews or knits or weaves, blends colors in a tapestry or creates a patchwork quilt, knows by the feel that a single thread is weak.*
>
> *But the weaving, the blending, the intertwining with the many others makes it strong.*
>
> *Any woman alone without friends to sustain her, to nurture and support, to hold with loving arms, like a single thread is weak.*
>
> *But the weaving, the loving, the nurturing of others, the networks of friendship makes her strong.*

(The Kinship of Women)

Merry Christmas to my tapestry of friends.

Center of the Universe

Is it possible that I am spoiled, foolishly living under the belief that the world does indeed revolve around me? Growing up, my siblings were oftentimes too quick to proclaim this as my most egregious flaw and the basis for my narcissism, and I am now pondering if maybe they were right and my sense of importance overinflated. It is interesting to me that the self-absorption that dominated my youth, which eventually diminished (somewhat?) as I matured into adulthood, may be taking center stage in my life again as I struggle with my illness. Do others who are facing such a health challenge fall into this trap, or am I really, at the heart of things, a self-centered brat? Geez, I was really hoping I was further along on my evolutionary journey than that.

My feelings were hurt Saturday night. I cried a little, cuddled up to my husband, and told him, like a pouting child, that my family hurt my feelings. I have not seen them in a couple of weeks as usual on our typical Saturday nights, and for a little while now, it seems the gatherings have become less than routine. Prior to this, I had become accustomed to my family being available, making me the center of attention, but mostly I adored having their love and support surround me, taking the energy they so willingly and unselfishly gave. So, I was very much looking forward to this past Saturday night and once again having everyone gather. But with the routine having become very "loose" lately, there didn't seem to be a sense of obligation from my family to commit, or worse yet, it didn't seem any of them considered that not gathering would be a huge letdown for me. And of course, I didn't tell anyone of the importance I had put on this particular Saturday night and my especially heightened anticipation, so how could they know? Except that it was my expectation, and I was disappointed.

Everyone had their reasons, all very valid. Mom wasn't feeling well. Rick and Ron were free at first, but then had to rearrange dinner plans with friends from Thursday to Saturday night—*my* night. Jeanette had semi-committed to joining me, but warned that Saturday was their only day to Christmas shop and get errands completed and that could potentially prevent them from coming over. Once that warning came to fruition, I knew she could hear the disappointment in my voice when she called to break the news. Michael was my sole savior that evening. And despite his welcome company, I could tell he was bored out of his skull without the interaction and distraction of other family members. (Chris and I are quite the entertaining pair these days.)

And this is why I am spoiled, because the disappointment is my own creation from my undisclosed expectations. I am sick and I miss them and it brightens my day when they are near me and with me. And I'm in the middle of my *last cycle*; I wanted them around to revel in that fact, to put me at the center of their universe again. I had been feeling relatively good, and I can't really guarantee that's how I'll feel in a few days on Christmas Eve, which is our next gathering, simply because of where I'll be in this final cycle. And this I (wrongly or rightly) thought trumped everything, yet I voiced this to no one. And it simply is not realistic to expect that I should be on their minds 24/7, while they have lives to lead, especially during the busy and stress-filled days of Christmas. Who can live up to that kind of expectation? And why should they? Particularly coming from me, a person already averse to asking for help—or anything, for that matter—and whenever I do, I feel I am imposing greatly on others (thanks, Mom).

So I pouted like a baby, and the further indication of my self-absorption and spoiled-brat status is that while the disappointment was real and acute, it didn't last long once I put my head on my husband's shoulder and he soothed away the hurt as if consoling a child. Or maybe the brevity of the pain really shows I am further along in my evolution than I thought. Yeah, right.

On a lighter and much happier note, I received my last in-office chemotherapy session today. Chris and his parents, who are in town for the holidays, joined me today for this monumental occasion and extolled words of excitement and encouragement. Strangely, I did not share their level of enthusiasm. I'm not sure if the day's significance hadn't registered or if I was erring on cautious optimism, or even a feeling that things are so routine and on their intended full-recovery path that the day felt anti-climactic. These feelings will probably sort themselves out in the coming days. And I'm fading fast this evening as I write this, surely due to low white blood cells (the latest count was nonexistent and I'm on house-arrest status again) and low platelets. I get a shot of Nesta tomorrow, and I anticipate needing platelets on Wednesday when I get another blood draw. Just a few more days of prednisone, my happy steroid, then the end of treatments is here. Thank goodness.

Trapped

And so this is Christmas—in the hospital. Just when I thought I was going to make it through this last round without complications, a last curveball is thrown my way, and I must learn again to expect the unexpected. I was pretty tired on Tuesday, having not slept well on Monday. I blamed it on my good friend prednisone and did not give much thought to how badly I was dragging, until around 8:00 that evening. I had been arguing with Chris since dinnertime. He was bothered by how I was not being respectful of him and his mother as they were trying to prepare food for me. And I was agitated that he would even go there with me in an already challenged position, but little did either of us know at that time how my capacity to deal with much of anything was being severely compromised by all the months of drugs and chemo, building steam against me, conspiring to throw me one last unforeseen challenge, ready to take me down. It cannot be comfortable in moments like these to be around a severely challenged ill person, one who looks like she can get around okay, and has for the most part been able to do basic things on her own, but then suddenly turns on a dime into a snippy, inconsiderate bitch. But that is what my husband and in-laws saw that night, and I had little concern for how that looked to anyone, knowing how crappy I was feeling. Pointing out the obvious misbehavior is not exactly how one should deal with a sick person in this state, and I was truly angry with my husband for not cutting me slack, for not understanding and walking a mile in my shoes. I scurried myself away upstairs to deal with my pity party and the two-inch-square box in which I felt myself trapped.

This is what it feels like when my body totally crashes: like I am stuffed inside a small box with windows, able to see what's going on around me, but unable to be fully present and rational, only this was to be the worst episode yet. I was angry for the state I found myself in, frustrated for the months the journey has been going on, and just so completely over it. It is not a time for rationality, for explanations; it is a time for letting me be. And I am sure that makes it excruciatingly hard for the healthy loved ones around me, but seriously, I didn't care, because I am sick and they are not. Unless I am driving real daggers into your body, don't take my words as if they are real daggers being driven into you. This is fucking hard.

And I was scared that night, too, because as the evening drew on, I could not release my anger, and together with the (unknown) infections growing inside me, it was not a good combination. Chris and I argued more in bed, and I could do nothing but scream and holler, pound my fists like exclamation points into our bed, the emotional meltdown complete. There was no capacity left, nothing, and he couldn't see it (nor could I see *him*—what this whole fucking mess has been doing to him). Until finally, his hand reached up to rub my back as he tried to pull me out of my suffocating box.

I had been feeling very lethargic all day, very much like I had felt when I had the staph infection two cycles ago, and my temperature was beginning to rise, but it was not yet a concern before bedtime. I didn't think I would be able to last through the night to get to a scheduled doctor's appointment in the morning for a routine blood draw. It terrified me to think I would find myself in the emergency room, and I dreaded the very real possibility that I could be spending Christmas in the hospital. I was spiraling, physically and emotionally. "No, this can't be," I cried. Chris was now very attentive and waking with me every hour (as if we could sleep) to check my temperature. My body continued to crash into discomfort. Around 1:30 am, my fever spiked to 101.6 and we called my doctor's office; thankfully, my doc was on call. Get to the ER, he said, and by 2:00 am, I was lying in a hospital bed, awaiting my fate.

By 5:00 am on the morning of Christmas Eve, I was admitted to the hospital. Initially, the medical team treating me thought I had a urinary tract infection, as I had complained of pain in my lower abdomen, on the left side above my pubic bone. This concern, along with nonexistent white blood cells, prompted the ER doctor, in consultation with my doc, to start me immediately on intravenous antibiotics. And that bought me a Christmas stay in the hospital. I tried eating a couple of hours later so I could take my oral prescription medication, but the pain on the left side of my abdomen worsened and I could barely eat my breakfast. The hospital floor doctor eventually ordered me pain medication so I could get some food in me and at least get the prednisone in my body—I still had six days left of this steroid to complete my last cycle.

Christmas Eve day was basically spent with me passed out with a fever, on pain medication, waking only a few minutes every hour to someone checking my vitals or talking in my room. The irony of it all: here I am almost free, the cancer surely (in my mind) eradicated from my body, yet on this last cycle, I feel the worst I have since my diagnosis. Because of the acute abdominal pain, a CT scan was taken, the results of which showed infection in both kidneys, more prevalent on the left side. Chris and his parents stayed with me most of the day, and a few of my family members stopped by early in the evening, as I was slowly starting to come around, but my mind was still really fuzzy and I didn't have much energy for visiting.

Today it is Christmas, and I awoke feeling much better, the constant drip of antibiotics starting to have some positive impact on my body. I was visited by more doctors in the morning: the floor doctor, an infectious-disease doctor, and my own doctor (who had also visited me yesterday). The source of the infection is still not known, but it is not the urinary tract, as they originally thought. Cultures have been taken of my blood and nothing has grown yet, so until they know the infection's origin, they will continue to treat me every six hours with intravenous antibiotics, which they have changed up a few times already in order to deliver the best coverage for what they think may be ailing me. This six-hour regimen makes it difficult to be treated on an outpatient basis, so it's unknown how many days I'll be here at this point.

And while it truly sucks to be spending the holidays here, I have to say it's been the best Christmas spent in the hospital ever. My wonderful husband brought Christmas to me. We have a miniature tree, which he dug out of our basement and delivered and set up in the hospital room last night. We also have a few Christmas cards taped to the wall. Chris stayed with me overnight, as he does during all my hospital adventures, and we played Christmas music all night as we slept. I was visited by many today, bringing me waves of Christmas love and joy. Chris's parents have been absolutely amazing, running back and forth to our house to bring us food and offering to do whatever it is we need. Their holiday visit has been interrupted, but they do not even think of it.

These are trying times, and I'm sure somewhere in the timing and struggle there is a higher meaning and purpose to it all. I haven't quite figured out what that is, but I'm sure some answers will be revealed once I ponder on that more when my brain is clearer. In the interim, the story I kept telling my family today is: fast-forward to 2009. It is Christmas, and Chris and I, along with our family members, are on a warm, tropical beach, all of us staying in a private villa, having earned this time together for the time robbed this year. It is my treat, my gift to them that we are there on that beach. This vision would not leave my mind, and I must find a way to make it happen, but probably not before I understand and pursue that higher purpose and meaning.

A Break in the Clouds

In the midst of winter, I found there was within me an invincible summer.

—Albert Careb

It is 1:30 AM and I am still in the hospital, unable to sleep, finding myself with a welcome dose of energy despite the early hour. My husband is sleeping soundly just five feet from me on the hard, uncomfortable couch, and I am listening to his sweet, gentle breathing and thinking how very lucky I am to have his love, to have this life.

I am happy to be crawling out of the mental pit of despair. My mind is a little clearer since this hospital adventure began, and I feel I am on a physical upswing. My white blood cells may finally be starting to multiply; we shall see in a few hours when they draw my blood. So, it is okay that I am wide awake at 1:30 writing this, as I can once again see the beauty of life inching closer to my soul and almost touch the sun-kissed sky, even as darkness drapes my room.

My infection is yet to be identified, and as of yesterday, with my counts still low (at less than 1 percent of what the body needs), the doctors still want to keep me here. Possibly later today they will identify the pesky little creature invading my body so they can narrow the specific antibiotic treatment that would enable me to go home and continue on an outpatient basis. I am encouraged that I have some energy now, even though it's the middle of the night. I think it is a good sign.

Chris will wake in a few hours to go home and gather his parents and take them to the airport. They have been troopers throughout this ordeal. His father is still challenged with a chronic foot injury suffered at work this summer, and his mother has been the rock for us this week, available to care for us in whatever capacity we needed. My family visited earlier in the day; it was good to see my sister and get my much-needed sister hug. She has this crook in her neck and chest where my head fits perfectly, and when she lets me rest there, her energy and love flow with full healing power from her heart and soul into mine.

Life is a challenge and a blessing. I know stronger days are ahead. I know in the midst of this winter, I will find within me an invincible summer.

The Finish Line

"I have to do what?" I asked my new doctor, an infectious-disease specialist, yesterday. He explained to me that I will be under his care for the next few weeks and he will have me continue on antibiotics for at least the next fourteen days—and I will need to administer this to myself intravenously at home. I was very uncomfortable with the idea.

My kidneys are infected with staph bacteria that may have been introduced through my port, although the doctor is not certain. The blood cultures taken several days ago were inconclusive, but because they were drawn after they had already started giving me antibiotics, the results are unreliable. And since I had the history of a staph infection in my blood two cycles before, the doctor suspects that the previous infection may not have cleared up completely. I will need to take at least two weeks of self-administered antibiotics, specific to this type of infection. Two to three weeks after this treatment, the doctor will do another blood culture to ensure the infection is gone. If it is not, he said, my port may indeed be the source and need to be removed. Generally, ports are left in one to two years after chemotherapy, in case of the unfortunate event of a relapse, but since I have completed my cycles, I am okay if my port needs to be removed. I won't miss it.

Yesterday, I was finally released from the hospital, after six days, the longest stay of the three hospital visits I've had since this journey began. Upon discharge, I was sent over to the infectious-disease office to learn how to give myself the daily antibiotics. Basically an access needle and tube are left in my port, and I'm supposed to first flush the port with a saline solution and attach a bag of antibiotics, let it drip for thirty minutes, then flush out my port when finished. I could opt to come in every day to the doctor's office for this procedure, but the doctor kept saying for the convenience factor, it's best to do it at home. I'm not sure whose convenience. I did okay with the lesson but was less than enthusiastic about having to do this by myself for several days.

This latest infection episode threw me for a loop, even more so than the internal hemorrhaging I had three months ago that sent me to the hospital for four days. Here it was my last cycle, and I could see the finish line. It's as if I have been running this long marathon, and the last mile has been the most difficult, the most painfully enduring. And I see the tape ahead of me, but before I reach it, someone comes from out of nowhere and body-slams me to the pavement. This scenario is played slow-motion in my mind, and as I am slowly but unexpectedly thrown off my feet and hurled to the ground, I let out a loud, bellowing, long-winded, "Noooooooooo!"

I am home now and so happy to be here. It has been a long and crazy ride for sure, full of twists and turns and highs and lows, but I have the rest of my life ahead of me. I am in full recovery mode. No more chemotherapy. No more prednisone. Sure, a couple of weeks of healing an infection, but that's nothing compared to how I felt last week. I do not know how long recovery will be; I'm told the steroids will take weeks to months to leave my body. Good riddance to this cancer, to 2008, and to a life that wasn't lived to its fullest potential.

POST-TREATMENT

A New Beginning

Slow Recovery
January 2009

When am I going to start feeling better? Is it too soon to expect just a little measurable improvement since being released from the hospital? Where is that corner I'm supposed to be rounding?

I had a follow-up appointment with the infectious-disease doctor this morning. I told him I've been feeling sort of blah the past few days, with muscle tenderness from going off prednisone. He explained to me that one of the side effects of the antibiotic is muscle soreness, but that is rare. He said he would check my blood counts and see if that's what is happening, but he said it's likely the prednisone. He wants me on twenty-one to twenty-eight days of antibiotics. When including the six days of treatment in the hospital, today is day ten, so I have eleven more minimum and as many as eighteen more days, administering drugs through my port at home. Now that I've learned how, I don't mind giving myself an IV bag of antibiotics—it's fairly easy. What I hate is having my port accessed with a needle 24/7 and having to cover up this patch with plastic and tape whenever I shower. This is a major inconvenience, and not only that, I worry about germs getting in the little tube that hangs from the needle. I just don't like it.

Once Chris and I got home today, I slept for a couple of hours. I awoke feeling pretty groggy, achy, and just out of it, as if I was coming down with a cold. I've been feverish since this afternoon and decided to call the infectious-disease doctor's office. I spoke with one of the nurses, who said to watch my fever, and if it hits 101, to go to the emergency room. It was at 100.3. I don't feel that great this evening, but it seems silly to me to go to the ER if my fever escalates. What are they going to do, anyway? I'm already on antibiotics. Give me Tylenol for the fever? I already took two, even though the nurse said not to. (She wanted me to let the fever run up if it was going to do that.) What else would they do, give me saline? I'll just drink more water. In any event, this late in the evening, I know I wouldn't get to see a specialist—they usually aren't around until morning—so why bother going to the ER? Having just spent six days and nights in the hospital, I really don't see the point of rushing myself there tonight, unless, of course, my symptoms get worse.

I just got off the phone with my brother Rick. He could hear in my voice how exhausted I am. And I am. Just so tired. I know it's only two days into the new year, *my year*, and I need to be patient. I just want to be free from this physical, emotional, and mental prison.

There were two parts to the overall seven months of treatment I received. The first half was cycles one through four, where I seemed to manage the treatments fine, with some surprising symptoms that, over time, I was able to manage. I certainly felt the physical challenge, but during the off week of each cycle, my level of energy truly rebounded. Then there was the second half, which began with the internal hemorrhaging in late September and culminated with this latest round of infection during my final eighth cycle. This half has kicked my ass. The physical teardown and the mental and emotional thrashing caught me off guard; there was very little in terms of energy recovery during the off weeks in between each cycle. My physical appearance changed the most, the weight gain was off the charts (more than thirty pounds), and I found it very hard to hold it together; my moments of inspiration came less frequently, and my love of life was waning. I'm still in this phase.

And so I ask again, when will I start feeling better?

And Now, the Icing on the Cake

Finally, it appears the corner arrived this morning, as I awoke feeling no pain, except a scratchy throat, and my mind a little more clear than it has been the past couple of weeks. A parting in the clouds, and as I took a step to round that corner—I hit a wall. That is, we hit a wall, Chris and I.

It was lunchtime and I was waiting on Chris to finish a business call so we could go out to eat when he walked into the room and told me to turn off the TV. "I just got let go," he said. We sat in silent disbelief as time stood still. Neither of us took a breath or blinked. We just looked at each other. A million thoughts swarmed my feeble mind in that brief moment. I am recovering from a major illness and we are both now unemployed. Smack! Big, tall, hard brick wall.

We are lucky. We are not destitute. As a couple, we have been good stewards of our money. We have very little debt and a healthy savings account, as we always had prudently believed our jobs could be vulnerable at our previous company. Yet, in the face of today's poor economic environment, where we both made the decision for me to quit my job and spend time on recovery and then develop a new career, Chris's new job could not survive the storm, and we find ourselves here. We both had talked about his getting laid off as a *possibility*, but we did not think it was a *probability*. This is life, and we are getting it in big, sobering doses.

So, let's recap: I have been through hell with this cancer; months of feeling ill until finally a diagnosis last summer, topped off by eight increasingly difficult rounds of chemotherapy with some medical emergencies thrown in for good measure; a difficult decision to not return to work; Chris with me every step of the way, quits his job to take a new, exciting, challenging position right as I get diagnosed; puts up with his sick wife for months, helps me through each of these cycles; sleeps in the hospital room through all the emergencies, including the six nights through Christmas, then the new year is here, *our year*, and he gets laid off. Are we being tested?

Chris is a highly talented and dedicated professional in his field, but he's also been restless since I've known him—always wondering if there wasn't something else he should be doing, another purpose to his life. Pre-illness, I had asked myself those same questions, but I wasn't restless; I had accepted my daily work, my career. Then, I got cancer, and yes, that was the big wake-up call to change the direction of my life. Maybe this is Chris's? The timing is curious.

New opportunities, Chris says, always the optimist. How else could we look at this situation, this past year? We are so blessed to have each other, our health (well, I'll get there), and in any given moment, there is no place we'd rather be than with each other, no matter the circumstance. He has been my rock, my biggest support through this difficult year, and often I wondered *who carried him*. He had enough strength for both of us. Now, as I recover, I may not be quite as solid as a rock, but I will be that strength for him. There's a lot of future ahead of us.

Road trip! That's what we were talking about earlier tonight, as we both have a lot of time on our hands right now. Or maybe a nice warm, tropical beach somewhere? We dreamed a little, then came back down to reality. We'll need to focus, put our heads together and prepare for all those new opportunities waiting for us. For now, I told him, today's a day for brownies, and I went about baking a pan. And now that they're out of the oven, we're going eat as many as we want. As Scarlett O'Hara infamously proclaimed, "After all, tomorrow is another day."

Searching for Solid Ground

When life hands you lemons, you make lemonade. Lemonade, in our case, is a trip to Hawaii! That's right, Chris and I are headed for the beach, just in time for our third wedding anniversary on Wednesday, and much-needed, well-deserved time away from all the madness and challenges from the past year, which was topped with the cherry of Chris's layoff several days ago.

Once my doctors gave the all-clear to travel this past week, we set about making our plans. Thank goodness for reward points earned on travel, business, and other purchases, which we have accumulated over the past couple of years—enough to allow us to book this vacation on the cheap. Chris and I were up until two this morning searching for the best way to spend these points. It was between Cancun and Hawaii, and the latter won out. Neither of us has ever been to Hawaii, so we look forward to experiencing the island together as virgins.

The shock from the news of Chris's job loss has worn off, although as this news continues to reach friends and family, we relive the reality of our current situation through their eyes. It is almost unbelievable. But here we are. We are grateful for the love and encouragement (and from some, the rage and disbelief) from family and friends. Chris has already made some good contacts from his vast business network and has a couple of leads he is exploring. We are both confident in his ability to find gainful employment soon. If only the economy—the worst yet since the Great Depression—would cooperate.

I have been an emotional basket case, and I am trying to pull myself together to be the support my husband needs right now. My emotions have ranged from anger to sadness to depression, as I felt the rejection of someone I love with all my heart and soul as if it were my own, and I took the layoff very personally. Thankfully, a couple of his ex-work cohorts called Chris to express their disappointment with the decision made to sever his employment, complimenting him on his contributions and work ethic. Once those calls were made, both Chris and I felt lifted and the pain from the loss was somewhat abated.

Despite this major setback in our lives, I do feel myself getting stronger each day. If only the outer shell of my body would start to reflect my inner recovery. In due time, Chris reminds me, be patient. I've been going to the gym with Chris the last few days. On the first day, my heart rate topped 150 beats per minute from just a ten-minute brisk walk on the treadmill! Today, I managed thirty-five minutes total on both the treadmill and elliptical machine (albeit on the equipments' lowest levels) and my heart rate exceeded 150 beats again. I have a way to go, but I am getting there. The fog that has been my brain's companion for months has almost all but dissipated; some lingering mists occupy corners of my mind, creating only momentary lapses of thought and concentration.

Recovery is here. Chris and I have each other. We have the love of friends and family. We're going to Hawaii. As the great Bob Marley sings, "Every little thing's gonna be alright."

Bookends and Beaches

We've been in the air now for an hour, and in just four more, the plane will touch down in Honolulu. My home, which has been the place of rest and recovery, has also been like a prison at times, and I feel like I have a week-long pass from jail. The last time I traveled was early June of last year, just days before ending up in the emergency room and receiving the cancer diagnosis. That trip was to a beach in Florida, and now I travel to a beach in Hawaii. These beach trips are like bookends on this road to health, the before and after, the awakening and journey to my soul.

Preparing for this trip was itself an adventure as Chris and I pulled out our summer clothes to pack. The journey of health recovery, coupled with the usual holiday eating frenzy, has left us both thick around the waist. Fortunately for Chris, he could find enough clothes to last him through our vacation, but unfortunately for me, nothing fit comfortably enough to fake it. *Those freakin' steroids*, I thought. Before letting me get thoroughly depressed and disgusted with myself, Chris quickly told me this is temporary and I just need to get temporary clothes. God, I love this man.

It was almost 8:00 pm, and off we went to Target and Kohl's, two great places for clothing life's temporary phases. We first stopped at Target, and after pulling multiple items off the clearance racks, I arrived at the dressing room and was met by a Target associate who was looking to coast through her last half hour of work and was clearly inconvenienced by my showing up with an armful of clothes to try on. "I'll be quick," I said with a smile, understanding her annoyance. She was neither pleasant nor helpful and retorted, "Well, you can only take six garments in at a time." I must have had more than twenty in my arms, and the whole process could have gone more quickly if a) she was nicer, and b) she allowed me to take all the garments in at one time. But no. *Humph*, I thought. I tried on a bathing suit (which thankfully didn't make me look like a beached whale) and left the dressing room—and my wig—to show Chris the outfit. The attendant caught sight of my bald head, and maybe she felt a little pang of guilt for her lack of customer service. Oops, did I do that on purpose—no, really?

Chris and I had the opportunity to meet up with friends prior to our tropical getaway. I had breakfast (of course!) with good friends Alex and Kristen and caught up with my BOTS girlfriends, whom I hadn't seen since our Christmas gathering. Later, both Chris and I met up with a handful of dear friends and ex-coworkers. It was fantastic to see them, most of whom I haven't seen since taking medical leave last June. They were delighted to see us and very kind and supportive with their comments. I am genuinely touched when I hear that people have kept up with me on my journal, and I am so humbled when they tell me how my entries, stories, and words have resonated with them or even inspired them to look at life differently, more openly. It warms my heart and makes my soul smile broadly.

Before taking this flight to Hawaii today, Chris and I flew in to San Francisco yesterday and stayed with my good friend Kim. I met Kim a few years ago when she lived in Colorado and became a member of BOTS. She works in the television industry as a writer/producer, and two years ago, when she was producing a program series about vacations, she asked if Chris and I would participate. We agreed and were featured in the program as a couple vacationing in New York—our fifteen minutes of fame. (Well, it was actually a full day of activity condensed to six minutes of airtime, displayed for all the world to see on cable television, so we really have nine minutes of fame left.) We had so much fun shooting with her, and I was in awe watching her at work. When we made our travel plans for Hawaii and saw that our trip connected us through San Francisco, there was no way we would miss the chance to see her.

Kim was working when we arrived, but she gave us directions to her apartment, which included stopping at the corner liquor store where she had left a key for us to pick up from the store owner, Lucky. From the airport, Chris and I took the BART (San Francisco's rapid transit system) close to her neighborhood and then a brief cab ride over to our predestined meeting with Lucky at the liquor store. It felt like we were on a covert operation. When Kim arrived home from work, we walked to a neighborhood restaurant. (SanFran boasts the most and the best neighborhood eateries; there are so many to choose from, it's hard to go wrong.) The conversation at dinner was lively and funny and sweet and sentimental as Kim shared with us her appreciation for my journal, which has allowed her to keep up with me during this time. A few tears were shed when she reached out for Chris's hand and thanked him for taking care of me through all of this; being away from Colorado had made her feel helpless, but knowing he was there by my side, she had great comfort and confidence that things would turn out fine. This touched my heart beyond words.

It was a hilarious scene this morning—and *so* Kim. Chris and I were up past midnight last night, and Kim was up even longer, so there wasn't much time this morning to get ready before taking us to the airport; she simply threw a robe on over her pajamas, slipped on her flip-flops, and away we went in her Mini Cooper. She pulled up to the airline drop-off area, got out of the car—robe, bed-head, flip-flops and all—and sent us away with the biggest hug before heading back home and back to her bed.

And now it is only a couple of hours before we land. Our beach vacation, where much rest and relaxation and life reflection will take place, hasn't yet started. But thirty-five thousand feet above the vast, blue Pacific Ocean, I find myself reflecting on these past several months and the enormity of it all, the great life transitions, the multitude of lessons I have learned (and have yet to learn), and the numerous gifts and blessings I have received. One important lesson or observation is that the universe (God, Higher Being, Mother Nature—all synonymous to me) is a partner in our individual plight, forever loving, forever giving, forever patient. It, He, She wants nothing more than our happiness and life's fulfillment and gives the gift of choice, free will, with which we decide how to experience and create this earthbound life. When we are negative, feel defeated, the universe waits patiently for us to decide otherwise, to change our direction and shift our perception. When our outlook is positive, when we take care of our bodies and minds, reach out to each other in genuine kindness and love, show no judgment and have more acceptance, live a kinder and gentler life, with full awareness and with our eyes wide open, the universe aligns with us and works with us, is no longer an observer from the sidelines, but rather a partner who opens up to us all things possible. It is timeless; it is joy and eternal love. And with this partner aligned with and gently guiding us, there is no challenge too great, no obstacle too difficult, no wall too high. I'm now ready for the beach. I'm ready to just *be*.

Resetting Our Souls

Six days have passed and we're back in the air again, a long flight back to San Francisco, leaving behind our beach holiday in Hawaii. Our first trip to the islands was part memorable, part forgettable, as I'm not sure Oahu and Waikiki were the perfect setting for our relaxing getaway. It was a nice trip overall, and we stayed at one of the top resorts on Waikiki Beach, but Honolulu is a thriving metropolis, crowded and quite expensive; they seem to "nickel and dime" you here (not that we're complaining, considering a good portion of this trip was paid for on travel points). The weather was cooperative half the time with sunshine and blue skies; we had rain and overcast skies the other half. I wish I were coming back with a golden tan; instead, I'm flying home with a miserable cold.

That's not to say Chris and I weren't grateful for this time away—we certainly needed it. We spent little time talking about our current situation, although I'm sure independently, we spent most of the time thinking about it. We rested as much as possible (two days of rain helped), despite the bustling international vibe at the resort and the large telecom convention taking place, which brought in hundreds of business travelers who made our wait for the elevators to and from our room excruciatingly long.

The sun, when it shone, was amazingly intense even for January, more intense than Colorado's summer sun. It felt nurturing and healing to bask in its glow. My recovery is limping along slowly; my energy is growing a little each day, and my mind is clearer. Chris even commented that the puffiness in my face is receding, although I can still see some swelling in my cheeks and my double chin is still present (maybe I can call it a chin-and-a-half at this point). The belly area seems to be retreating some, too, as I can now see my toes when I look down at my feet. The hair is certainly taking its sweet little time to grow back; although I feel peach fuzz on my head, still not much is going on there.

Airports are great indicators for how in shape you are. Carting around luggage, walking forever to gates and baggage-claim areas, stowing bags above and below your seat—all these activities for a recovering cancer patient are a major workout, raising my heart rate, putting me out of breath, with my body breaking out in sweats. I had packed workout clothes with the intention of utilizing the resort's gym, but those clothes never got worn, as I never made it to a workout. Vacationing—the getting here, that is—wore me out, and with the onset of a cold halfway through the trip, well, there just wasn't much energy left to pay homage to a treadmill.

Chris and I did enjoy walks on the beach and lying out in the sun, and the local cuisine. Yesterday, we rented a car and toured the circumference of the island. Oahu is gorgeous with incredible vistas, towering lush, green mountains, and beautiful beaches, some with a wicked surf, others with a docile, more tranquil, turquoise water caressing the sandy shoreline. The vegetation is fascinating and curious, large banyan trees with outstretched limbs, and in some places, we saw pine trees with branches that looked sparse in comparison to the pine trees on the mainland, but up close, the branches had large, long needles stretching upward toward the sun. "They look like thick eyelashes," I commented to Chris. Many of the island's homes and buildings were built in the late fifties to seventies, with little modern building since. Honolulu is the exception, where it appears they are either erecting a new high-rise or renovating one every week.

While we will miss our little island getaway and the distance it put between us and our recent challenges, we are somewhat anxious to get home to the comfort and familiarity of our house and our bed and to see what life has in store for us—or rather, what we have in store for life.

Stuck in the Mud

Tired and uninspired is how I've been feeling the last few days since arriving home from Hawaii. I thought the time away and different scenery would take the edge off reality and put me in a better mental place. Maybe it did for a little while, but I must admit I've been feeling a little blue lately. Part of it is this darn cold I have, which seemingly wants to hang around and is dragging me down physically. And now I've given it to Chris, so the two of us have been hacking up a lung for the past couple of days. It's difficult to find energy and inspiration to alter the course of your life when your head is thick with congestion and your ears are ringing. And it's so cold outside. I just want to lie in bed all day long, sheltered by my warm bed and comforter, and forget about all our worries. But our jobless situation and my very s-l-o-w recovery are nagging at my brain, giving me the blahs. I just need to give myself a break, really. At least until I get over this cold and have the strength to face these issues.

Chris is out of town on a job interview. The position is in the same industry he was in, and the role is similar as well, except the job isn't here. I haven't been able to wrap my brain around the prospect of living someplace else, far away from my family-and-friend network, especially given that my head is about to explode anyway. And that makes it difficult to be an enthusiastic support for my husband, which he needs and deserves. Of course I absolutely support him; it's just the enthusiasm is a matter of degree. He does have some connections and prospects here at home; unfortunately, they are less developed than this out-of-state opportunity. I pick him up from the airport in a couple of hours, and we'll have much to talk about, I'm sure.

I haven't done much about my new career, either. The manuscript (my journal) has been printed and ready for my editing, but it sits there, unworked. The agents I was to contact have yet to be contacted. The research I was supposed to continue has yet to be continued. Again, I just need to give myself a break. I'm still recovering, and even though the roller coaster from the past treatments has smoothed out to a more even ride, the pace is unbearably slow. Patience. My life's biggest lesson. I mean, we just got back a few days ago, for goodness' sakes. I've had seven loads of laundry and two doctors' appointments, and Chris is out of town on an interview in that timeframe. All of this with a miserable cold. Why can't I just chill? Take a deep breath.

I go NPO tonight at midnight, nothing by mouth (how NPO translates to "nothing by mouth" I am not sure—shouldn't it be NBM?), as I have a bone marrow biopsy procedure scheduled tomorrow morning. My doctor can perform this procedure in his office, but I have no desire to be under a local anesthetic and hear a drill pierce my body and grind through bone—no, thank you. Luckily, I had the option to have this done under general anesthesia at the hospital. I'll be groggy and out of it for a few hours after the procedure tomorrow. Maybe I'll find some inspiration and a better attitude, as I seem to do better under the influence of (legal) drugs—odd, isn't it? I only hope this won't be a necessary crutch going forward in my new career. Unless I can convert that crutch to a bottle of red wine shared with good friends, or, of course, my darling husband. That would be alright.

The two doctor appointments I had were follow-ups with my oncologist and the infectious-disease guy. Both went well. My blood counts are stabilizing and improving: white blood cell counts at 5.1, hemoglobin at 10.9, and platelets finally rebounding to 83. There is still a ways to go with the hemoglobin and platelets, but these numbers are good and the reason for my more even ride. The staph infection seems to be cured at this point, and the infectious-disease doc will not do a blood culture unless my oncologist decides to leave my port in. I discussed with my oncologist my wish to have it removed, and he didn't have an issue with that. The only reason it would be left in is if the test results from the bone marrow biopsy and PET scan (scheduled in a couple of days) aren't clear or conclusive, which is not what we expect. The end to all the treatments, procedures, and multiple doctor appointments is coming. Only a couple more weeks and I will be home-free and singing, "Cel-e-bration time, come on!"

Doubts and Fears

I am only days away from what I expect to be one of the happiest moments of my life, and yet I have been spending the past several days in a deep funk. Why is it that as I sit on the precipice of freedom, at the top of the mountain ready to proclaim my victory over cancer, I am feeling so depressed? The morose feelings and sadness are truly profound and seem so out of place right now.

As the clouds part in my brain, and a blue sky paints across my mind's canvas, I am becoming woefully aware of my existence, my being, and I don't see the maturation, the altruistic vision I had for myself at this point in my journey. And I am deeply disappointed with myself. The old patterns of thought, the "me" I am so familiar with but was so anxious to trade in for a more evolved being, has returned. And I realize I don't like her. It seems incredibly self-serving and narcissistic to appear to be ungrateful for arriving at this spot—surely cured—and to not appreciate myself for the struggle and journey. Particularly when so many others who have battled cancer lost the fight, did not get to where I am right now, did not get the chance to hear their doctor tell them they are in remission. Do I feel guilty? Better yet, unworthy? Are these feelings normal?

Tonight, Chris and I had a discussion about his pending job prospects, and the realistic possibility that the out-of-state opportunity could come to fruition. He told me he didn't feel I supported him and that I wasn't ready to commit to a move. I was pretty defensive of his observation. After I gave my surface explanation about how I am a pragmatist and I am only looking at this opportunity with much caution and questioning whether it is the right move for us right now, but that I surely support him, I came to the root conclusion that I am scared, and that I doubt whether I can physically handle a move. I have lost much confidence in myself and my abilities. I have lived for more than a year being less than who I had been; I am no longer certain of what I can commit to and whether I can show up to the task at hand.

Recognizing the defeat in my voice and hearing my self-doubt, Chris came to my rescue and acknowledged my pain. He told me to give myself a break, and that all he wants me to do is focus on getting better. Let him focus on finding the job and making our home and our lives secure, he said. He held me, let me cry on his shoulder, and wiped the tears from my eyes. My knight in shining armor, on his white horse, holding his damsel in distress. He helped slay my dragons of fear and insecurity (for now), and in the process helped me find my motivation and inspiration again.

I must quiet my mind and find peace, so that I can then tend to a greater purpose than myself. This is where I want to be, but I need to show up with my heart and soul whole and ready to shine a light unto the world. Be. Still. Know. I. Am.

Cancer-Free

February 2009

I've been waiting eight long months for this day. Today, I am in remission. Today, I am a Cancer Survivor! How sweet the victory, how bright the sunshine. Victory and sunshine—two keys to my soul and my journey.

There will be no false alarm this time. My doctor thoroughly reviewed the test results and was prepared for our meeting. He was happy to deliver such great news, with a bit of caution that I appreciated and welcomed. Nothing is guaranteed; life is not on automatic pilot. Both the bone marrow biopsy and PET scan results showed no indication of cancer, and nothing from the reports caused him any concern, not even the inflammation around a lymph node under my right armpit. I had reported to him some tenderness I was feeling in that area during my last meeting with him, thinking it might be an ingrown hair, and apparently that inflammation showed up on the scan. It didn't concern him. Still, his tone was conservative and his conclusion was cautious. Was he unsure? My guess is that he, too, understands that there are no guarantees. And that while the reports say one thing, life can always dictate otherwise. There are no falsehoods here, no overassumptions. Just the facts, ma'am. And that is good enough for me.

I was in such emotional pain last night, on the eve of this great day. Chris and I first engaged in a civil, productive discussion about the appropriate direction of our lives, but this gradually escalated into an argument and fight, each one of us exhausted from the journey of my illness and nervous over our current predicament; neither one of us giving the other the proper support and understanding that was obviously needed and sadly denied. Last night, which was supposed to be spent in giddy anticipation, was spent in turmoil and then silence as we went our separate ways, angered and hurt by the words spoken and unspoken. I wept in bed alone, scared about the future, pissed at the missed opportunity for joyful calm the evening could have been, wondering about the stranger whom I'd married. I reached for Amber to help me sleep. I did not hear Chris come to bed.

When I awoke this morning, the awful feelings that accompanied me to sleep were there to greet me as I groggily opened my eyes. The punishing emotional silence continued for a couple of hours until we were in the elevator on our way to my doctor's appointment. There, in a confined eight-by-eight-foot space with no windows to capture our gaze, there was no room for tension, anger, or hurt, and we could not help but glance in each other's direction until finally our eyes met—his big, green, and beautiful, and mine achingly saying I needed reassurance and love. Chris pulled me close and kissed my forehead and said, "We're going to be alright." In that moment, we were a unit again, made whole in a matter of seconds on an elevator going up only one floor, ready to hear the anticipated good news from my doctor.

After hearing the freeing words of all-clear from the oncologist, I asked him a barrage of questions:

"With my white blood cell count at 3.6, should I be concerned?"

"You will have white blood cell counts on the low end of the range the rest of your life."

"Is that a concern?"

"No."

"Am I in menopause permanently, or will my reproductive cycle return?"

"Yes, I believe it will return for you."

"What happens if the disease comes back? Is another round of chemotherapy the treatment protocol, and will my body be recovered enough to take it?"

"I don't believe it will come back, but, if it does, no, chemotherapy is not the treatment. Regardless of how recovered you are from that, the next step, should it be necessary, is a bone marrow transplant. We would want to introduce all new healthy cells into your body."

"What is the next step going forward?"

"I want to see you monthly and monitor you closely."

"For how long?"

"Indefinitely. I mean, for probably a few months. Then we'll go to every couple of months, eventually every few months, etc."

I confirmed with him that I wanted my port removed, and we discussed my heart rate, which continues at a high, steady pace. He said this will eventually come down, but upon concern expressed from Chris, he decided to order a MUGA scan of my heart. Both procedures will be scheduled in the coming days. After that, monthly follow-up appointments and all is well with the world.

Chris and I left the office, full of renewed spirit and life. We went to Lucille's to celebrate with a Bloody Mary and late breakfast (of course).

Technology is amazing nowadays, with the various ways to keep in touch with friends and family and the speed at which you can get a message out. I sent phone text messages to many and received instant replies to our good news. Once home, I posted a note on Facebook (a.k.a. "Crackbook") and reached many others through that medium. The news seemingly spread like wildfire as dozens of friends and family members reached out to me and Chris in kind.

Tonight, Chris arranged an impromptu dinner out with family members. My sister and three of her daughters, along with Michael and his daughter, and Rick and Ron, joined us to celebrate. It was the first time I went out in public baring my quasi-bald head, which is now sprouting tiny black hairs all over the once-smooth, shiny surface. I still look bald—it just looks like my head is dirty. But I didn't care—it was a night to celebrate.

What an amazing day it has been. Hell, what an amazing journey it has been and continues to be. And tonight, as I write this, I am sitting on the leather chaise lounge in the sanctuary my husband created for me eight months ago. I have not journaled from this spot in many, many weeks. Once I was feeling better and mobile, I preferred writing on my laptop in a variety of places in my home, at the doctor's office receiving chemo, or in the hospital receiving blood. Still, this retreat has served me well, giving me a place for respite and tranquility early on. It has been a place for healing, a warm bear hug when my body was frail and my mind weary and foggy. Like an old, loyal friend, it has comforted me through my weakest moments as a person sick with cancer; now it cuddles and holds me up proudly as a *Survivor*. It has been everything my husband envisioned it would be for me.

And as I sit here in the comfort of my retreat, I am reveling in the words written, the voice messages left by friends and family who have been with me each step of the way. Many of whom I have kept in close contact with, and many more of whom I am surprised to find out have continued to keep abreast of my progress. There can be no doubt that all the positive energy from these wonderful souls, together with their calling upon God, or their chosen Higher Being, has had a part in my healing. *For I know I was carried in my darkest hours of physical pain and mental anguish and brought safely to this place in time by some force greater than my sheer determination to be well.*

Humility, my good friend, has joined me again, and I cannot wait for the next chapter of my life to begin.

All the World's a Classroom

Recovery is going well. The body is an amazing thing. I have been exercising almost daily the past couple of weeks since getting over my cold, and each day, I am encouraged by my progress. I have the giddiness of a baby who delights at the accomplishment of taking his first steps whenever I push myself to the next level of physical exertion. I am still far from my body's fitness of one and a half years ago, but at least now I can see the possibility of its return in the not-too-distant future.

Slowly, the effects of the steroid prednisone are leaving my body, and I am starting to recognize my face in the mirror as the puffiness is receding. I still have much of the excess weight around my middle section, having dropped only a few pounds since being home from my Christmas hospital stay. This has me somewhat disappointed, as I got used to the small frame the disease left me with prior to being diagnosed. But that was an unhealthy, slimmer me thirty pounds ago. At my current weight, I am only about ten pounds over my normal weight before all this began. And I'm not sure that the weight I have gained can be referred to as healthy either, considering it was mostly drug-induced. In due time, I keep telling myself, I will get to that elusive healthy, happy state.

I took a couple of days off from the workout regimen this past week, as I had two final procedures performed. The MUGA scan tests the heart's efficiency, and from my research, I discovered that it is typically given at the beginning, midpoint, and end of chemotherapy treatment. I am not sure why my doctor did not order this exam for me before now, except that it is possibly optional at the beginning if there is no prior history of heart problems. I asked the technician if the scan would indicate why my heart rate is high, and he said no. It is only testing the heart's strength to determine if there was any damage from the chemotherapy. I asked him what if there was damage, and he said my doctor would probably order up another test in a month, allowing more time for the heart to recover. He didn't seem too concerned if the test came back with a low efficiency reading. Regardless, I have been feeling good and would be surprised if I have any issues with my heart, considering I have been able to steadily increase my level of physical activity without undue stress.

The other procedure I had that same day was the removal of the port in my chest. The nurse who last assisted with the procedure of inserting my port was the same one who attended to me for the removal, and she remembered me. I continue to be impressed that these caretakers remember their patients, even eight months later. I, too, remembered her because I commented last time that she reminded me of Scarlett Johanssen. She said no one had ever told her that. As I was being prepped for surgery, I told her that there had to have been more than a hundred procedures and patients she tended to in the last eight months and I was surprised she remembered me. She told me that on the days ports are inserted, many patients are sad or apprehensive about the health issues they face, and when they come back for its removal, then those are happy days because it almost always means they are cured. Not everyone comes back as quickly (*if at all*) as I did for a port removal, and that's why she remembered me. The procedure went well, and I am only a little sore at the incision area.

Hair has been interesting. It's growing back slowly. Each time I look in the mirror, I think of how a watched pot never boils. Well, a watched bald head never grows hair. I've got some measurable amount of peach fuzz sprouting up there, but the basic look is still "bald." I am just wondering, *When will it all return?* And I'm beginning to notice the very fine, delicate hairs that cover our bodies, which I've never noticed before now. They are sprouting all over my body and I swear, as a healthy person, I never paid any attention to them. But there they are—on my forehead, on the sides of my face and cheeks, on my neck and lower back; tiny, blonde, and silky. I notice them now because for months, I've had nothing but a slippery, smooth surface of skin. It's weird, I tell you.

It's been almost two weeks since I've written here in my journal, the longest lapse between entries since this journey began. I have been absent and contemplative these several days as Chris and I have tried to gain a footing in the circus of the unemployed. To say we have seen eye to eye on our next steps would be a gross overstatement, and many of the past few days have been painful as we have tried to navigate these uncharted waters, which is testing the strength of our marriage. Going through this as a healthy adult is challenging enough; wandering through the quagmire as a recovering cancer patient is especially grueling. Thankfully, the past couple of days have found us coming together on the same page, in much-needed support of one another and in recognition of the importance of our union. We are calmer about our current state. Each day, we grow more confident about our prospects, and every moment, we are stronger in our commitment to each other.

I continue to be a student in the subject of life. Most of the time, I am an active participant; other times, I am a casual observer; sometimes I am a know-it-all; and on occasion, I am a rebellious student. The lessons are always valuable but sometimes difficult. But mostly, I am grateful for the chance to sit in the classroom and learn that, though I don't have all the answers, I can make out of the subject what I please through my own creativity and free will. There are no right or wrong answers, only potential for growth and a certainty of continued lessons. For this course of life never ends, and suddenly I see this is where I want to be.

Take Me Home

March 2009

Almost heaven—West Virginia. Life's next challenge is here, and we are moving. Chris accepted a job with a company located in West Virginia, *mountain momma.* I have been reticent to journal during the past few weeks, not sure how to assess, dissect, or manage the whipsaw of emotions heaped on my shoulders, eventually settling in the pit of my stomach. What kind of universe kicks me down with cancer, pulls me into survival, and then orders me to leave my comfort zone, my beautiful Colorado?

Of course, I am not in this alone. Never have been. My wonderful husband has been at my side, and the view from his saddle has been much different than mine, even though we occupied the same space, the same circumstance of my illness and recovery, his layoff, and now his new venture. And together, it is our next adventure. We have arrived at this point in time, intact, although neither of us will ever fully comprehend what the other went through to get here. There have been three journeys: his, mine, and ours. And it is the latter that prevails; it is that path which matters most.

During the past month, we traveled to the South to visit family and friends and for Chris to reconnect to his network of past work colleagues and bosses, anything to drum up opportunities for employment. (He used to live and work in Atlanta.) We weren't sure if the West Virginia opportunity would pan out, and it made sense to explore other options in addition to the contacts he was making in Colorado. It was during our trip that he received the call and offer from the company located in the Appalachian state, and we spent a couple of soul-searching, gut-wrenching (mostly my gut was wrenching) nights discussing the matter. Chris was truly excited about the position; I was mentally a million miles away hiding in the comfort of my *own* mountain state with three hundred days of sunshine. But the weight of the current economic climate was too heavy for us to toss aside, and for now, this is the best direction for our journey to travel.

So back home we came to ready our house to sell. I hate the process of moving. It is a pain. And trying to get motivated for an already stressful process is that much more difficult when my emotions are gripping at my heart and wanting me to stay put. This reality against the backdrop of my recovery has been a bit overwhelming—but not insurmountable. I mean, I just survived cancer, for God's sake. And while I would rather just be given a break and coast into my next adventure, the truth is I went through that horrible ordeal and survived—I think I can handle this bump in the road.

Feeling sorry for myself is also something I hate. So before I send out invitations to my pity party, I need to remind myself how lucky and blessed we are. Millions are suffering without a job right now, not knowing how they'll keep their houses or feed their families. My father-in-law was laid off just this week from a company where he has spent the majority of his working life. My good friend from junior high school, whom I recently reconnected with, is in town to hold vigil at her dying mother's bedside. My dear cousin, who sadly had to put her cat down yesterday, accompanied her husband to a doctor's appointment today to determine if he potentially has a very serious illness. My brother-in-law continues his fight with MS and is trying to find the right medication to slow a disease for which there is no cure. Life doesn't always bend in our favor; it throws curveballs and sometimes lobs grenades—no one is immune. But there is hope. There is love. There is joy. These things abound eternally, and this is where we find solace, comfort, peace from the crazy detours in life—when we choose them.

I will be closer to my extended family in our new home. I have been thinking about my aunts, uncles, and cousins the past couple of weeks, wanting to reach out to them with the great news, except I knew my enthusiasm wouldn't yet meet theirs, so I procrastinated, waiting for the right timing and emotional lift. Just as I was building up to a sustained level of quasi-excitement, my cousin Conni sent me an e-mail checking in on me. Out of the blue. So I wrote her back to tell her of the latest news, that we will be neighbors, within only a two-hour drive from her. And later that same afternoon, I got a call from my Aunt Kathryn. Out of the blue. I asked her if she had talked to Conni (suspecting that may be the reason for her call); she said no, and that I had been on her mind. So I gave her the news, that Chris and I would be neighbors to her (two hours in the other direction from my cousin). She was ecstatic and giddy with excitement. News spread, and I began hearing from other family members out east. I will literally be living in the middle of them all—there in the center, a place I have seemingly been occupying for several months now.

Chris started his new job this week (just as his father lost his). I am continuing to prep our house and get it ready to sell. We've been talking several times a day, and I miss him dearly. He'll be home this weekend, then gone again, this time for two weeks. I'll join him during his next trip out, and together, we'll traverse the landscape to find our next home, which will likely be a transitional one before we decide to invest in something more permanent. I'll have a few more weeks of my beautiful Colorado and all its warmth and sunshine, and, of course, all my wonderful family and friends. Life is bittersweet.

My former boss and good friend visited me yesterday. I updated him on our latest pending venture and the angst and emotions I was experiencing, which has quieted my quill. He told me—inspired me, really—to keep writing, saying that I have a voice and a message for so many. He explained to me that not many people have been through my experience with cancer, but many more have been where Chris and I are right now, facing a new job, a new move. Write about that, too, he said. And so I have found my pen again, and my voice. And once again, I am facing the sun, with arms outstretched, ready for our new adventure to begin and for the chance to let my soul sing.

West Virginia, mountain momma, take me home.